# HAVEN'T YOU
# SUFFERED
# ENOUGH?

## CLINICALLY PROVEN METHODS
### *to* CONQUER STRESS

# HAVEN'T YOU SUFFERED ENOUGH?

## CLINICALLY PROVEN METHODS
### *to* CONQUER STRESS

## DR. BRENDA LYON, PhD, CNS, RN

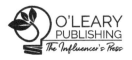

O'LEARY
PUBLISHING
*The Influencer's Press*

BONITA SPRINGS, FL

Published in the United States by
O'Leary Publishing
www.olearypublishing.com

The views, information, or opinions expressed in this book are solely those of the authors involved and do not necessarily represent those of O'Leary Publishing, LLC.

This book does not give medical advice. The content of this book is not meant, in any manner, to replace the care of a physician or other medical provider.

ISBN: 978-1-952491-00-9 (print)

ISBN: 978-1-952491-01-6 (ebook)

Library of Congress Control Number:  2020907565

Book Design by Jessica Angerstein
Editing by Heather Desrocher, Jessica Jones and Matthew Acton

## DEDICATION

I dedicate this book to my family, my mother (who is ninety-seven years old), my three fabulous brothers and their wives, my nieces, nephews and great nieces and nephews. They are continually supportive of me in more ways than I can enumerate.

As this book goes to print, all who are not essential workers are hunkered down in their homes to help flatten the curve of the COVID-19 virus that is taking a devastating toll on our country. So, additionally, I dedicate this book to all of the dedicated health care professionals, support staff, first responders, truckers and food supply staff who are courageously confronting exceptionally difficult situations daily.

# CONTENTS

Foreword ............................................................................................... ix

Preface ................................................................................................. xi

Acknowledgements ............................................................................ xv

Introduction ......................................................................................... 1

**CHAPTER 1**   Rethinking Stress ............................................................ 11

**CHAPTER 2**   When Demands and Resources Are Out of Balance .................... 35

**CHAPTER 3**   Eliminating Non-essential Demands ................................ 59

**CHAPTER 4**   Maximizing Resources ................................................... 87

**CHAPTER 5**   How You Perceive Difficult Situations ........................... 107

**CHAPTER 6**   Conquering Dysfunctional Anxiety ................................ 129

**CHAPTER 7**   Conquering Unjustified Guilt ........................................ 151

**CHAPTER 8**   Conquering Chronic Anger ........................................... 167

**CHAPTER 9**   Conquering Frustration ................................................. 193

**CHAPTER 10**  Dealing With Loss, Grief and Situational Depression ................ 203

Epilogue ............................................................................................ 221

Quick Guide: TIPS to Prevent and Eliminate Stress ........................... 223

References .......................................................................................... 227

About the Author .............................................................................. 237

# FOREWORD

Physicians rarely read the nursing literature. I think this is in large part due to time constraints and the near impossibility of keeping up with their own published specialty research. Dr. Lyon's book is a must read for all physicians, caregivers and providers who struggle with caring for patients who have stress-based illness.

I was privileged to read the preprint version of this book. I learned so much that I was never taught in medical school or in post-graduate continuing medical education. This book is very logical and based on sound theory and research; moreover, it is loaded with self-help tips to help the reader cope when feeling very overwhelmed with the reality of their daily work and social life.

Dr. Lyon draws on over 30 years of experience as a stress management counselor to share engaging, real-life stories of clients she has worked with, as well as her own personal experience, to offer practical strategies in both preventing and eliminating stress. Dr. Lyon's work is for all clinicians who would like to add its rich content to their own practice tactics in helping those who think and feel they are at their wits' end and manifest somatic complaints of stress-based illness. These unfortunate patients represent a large majority of primary care practice. My own practice, in cancer genetics, creates information that some patients find extremely difficult to deal with and, in response, experience extreme and dysfunctional anxiety and unjustified guilt. This book will soon be added to the various tools I provide to assist patients in coping with stress and anxiety. *Haven't You Suffered Enough?* is a must read for health care professionals and the lay public!

Glenn Jay Bingle, MD, PhD, MACP
Medical Director: Genetic Services and Counseling Community Health Network & Clinical
Professor of Medicine, Medical and Molecular Genetics
Indiana University School of Medicine
Indianapolis, Indiana

# PREFACE

Although most of us need little introduction to the experience of stress, we've desperately needed a sound theoretical and research-based explanation of the phenomenon with practical strategies to both prevent and eliminate it. The self-care skills taught in *Haven't You Suffered Enough?* can go a long way in preventing and eliminating the suffering and negative health effects that result from prolonged stress in what can be a demanding world.

All of us experience difficult or challenging circumstances, all of which can be fertile territory for the experience of stress. What if the majority of people really understood stress and the controllable factors that can be changed to both prevent and eliminate it, despite difficult circumstances? How much more effectively would we be able to function as individuals? How much more would our society thrive?

On the physiological level, the experience of stress triggers the release of stress hormones by the adrenal glands. In the short term, these responses may be adaptive because they produce an emergency reaction, which may allow for more effective coping in avoiding or altering a dangerous situation. However, the prolonged experience of stress results in the overall decline of the body's biological functioning because of the continued secretion of stress hormones. Over time, the physiological impact of stress can cause a deterioration of body tissues, such as blood vessels and the heart. We are learning more about how stress can alter our immune systems as well. In addition to these major health difficulties, many of the minor aches and pains we experience may be caused or worsened by stress. These include headaches, backaches, skin rashes, indigestion, fatigue, diarrhea and constipation, as well as the possibility of a whole class of psychosomatic disorders.

On a psychological level, high levels of stress prevent people from coping with life adequately. Their view of the environment can become clouded, and, in extreme cases, some people are unable to act at all. Moreover, people can become less able to deal with new difficult situations. *The ability to contend with future stress then declines as a result of past stress that has accrued and been unresolved. This can manifest in many ways, such as inter-personal conflicts and unhappy relationships.*

All these consequences then beg the question, how *can* we most effectively cope with stress? Are there guidelines and strategies that have been proven effective? Are there internal and external resources we can tap and summon? Thankfully, the answer to these questions is *yes*, and *Haven't You Suffered Enough?* contains these answers, and many others, all of which can be useful both for mental health professionals looking to help clients manage their stress, as well as the lay person who may be looking for guidance about how to skillfully prevent and eliminate stress in their lives. Thus, this book functions well in both personal and academic settings.

In addition to covering long-standing strategies such as emotion-focused and problem-focused coping, *Haven't You Suffered Enough?* explores how balancing our demands and resources and controlling our thoughts can lead to preventing and eliminating the stress emotions. *Haven't You Suffered Enough?* carefully and systematically teaches the reader how to reframe difficult situations as challenges, how to reduce the perceived threat of a stressful situation, and how and why to develop a more beneficial relationship with your thoughts. Fundamentally, *Haven't You Suffered Enough?* helps the reader gain a resilient mindset to both prevent and eliminate stress.

By using powerful stories, personal vignettes, observations born from research and decades of clinical experience, and the best scientific knowledge available, *Haven't You Suffered Enough?* thoroughly shows the reader how to get a grip on both preventing and eliminating stress. In fact, *Haven't You Suffered Enough?* proves to be both theoretically sound and immensely practical. Each step, each skill, and each insight is broken down into its most fundamental parts, making this an easy-to-read and easy-to-apply prescription for daily living. More specifically, the reader receives detailed instruction for how to:

1. Balance demands and resources by eliminating non-essential demands and maximizing resources,
2. Proactively manage how you view difficult situations,
3. Disempower negative thoughts and empower positive thoughts,
4. Find and maximize one's capacity to control difficult situations, and
5. Effectively deal with anxiety, guilt, anger, frustration and grief, as well as situational depression.

The experience of reading this book mirrors what it would be like to be in a session with Dr. Lyon. The straightforward exercises included in *Haven't You Suffered Enough?* demystify stress and provide new and inspired leadership in the field of mental health resources. The nature of stress requires, from all of us, continued improvement, and new paths of innovation, awareness, and preparedness, and this text provides just such a roadmap. And, since treating professionals and caregivers, especially, need to understand the entire continuum of care, and the unique role their chosen role plays, silo-knowledge is insufficient. Treating stress is an interdisciplinary exercise. To successfully treat stress, one must consider and treat the whole person: the physical, cognitive, psychological, interpersonal, and spiritual aspects of being. *Haven't You Suffered Enough?* shows the reader how to do precisely that. It's not often that you find a book that can serve as a practical book for the lay public and as a text for use in the academic setting.

Nate Hinerman, PhD, Licensed Marriage and Family Therapist (LMFT)
Associate Professor
Department Chair, Psychology
Undergraduate Studies, Golden Gate University
San Francisco, CA

# ACKNOWLEDGEMENTS

I'm grateful to so many who have contributed to my career, including Indiana University School of Nursing. The School supported me in multiple ways as I was working to develop my expertise in my specialty area of stress and stress-related illness. A big thank you goes out to Dr. Victoria Champion and Dr. Pat Ebright as reviewers of early drafts.

I also want to thank each and every private client (whose names are changed in the text) with whom I've had the privilege to work. They taught me so much, as we worked together to eliminate their stress-related illnesses.

I'm so very grateful to Jessica Dorfman Jones, my editor. She pushed me to simplify my language, asked great questions to help me clarify particularly complex concepts, and made wonderful suggestions for organizing the content. She is the BEST!

I also want to recognize and thank the O'Leary Publishing team. Specifically, Heather Desrocher and Mathew Acton for meticulous copy and line editing and Jessica Angerstein for top-notch design work. They were great!

If you are experiencing troublesome symptoms and think you might be experiencing a stress-related illness, it is important that you see your physician to rule out any possible causes of your symptoms that would require medical treatment. This book does not give medical advice. The content of this book is not meant, in any manner, to replace the care of a physician or other medical provider.

# INTRODUCTION

I always wonder about the author's backstory when I am reading a book. Assuming you might feel the same way, here's the story of how I developed a passion to understand stress emotions and stress-related physical illness and then treat them. Within that story is another important tale, how I developed the practice and the techniques that I share with you throughout the book. In my work with clients, I learned the common causes of stress emotions and how to both prevent and alleviate them.

As with every good story, this one starts with people. In this case, the people are me and my fellow high school students. When John F. Kennedy was assassinated in 1963, I was in Latin class when we learned his fate. I felt very sad, some of my classmates were afraid, some were angry, and most were just stunned. I also experienced anger later that day, but our initial responses were quite varied in response to the same event. Since that day, I have been intrigued by human emotions. I remember being amazed at how many of us could experience the same event yet react with very different emotions. That moment shaped my entire career.

## SAME DISEASE, DIFFERENT EXPERIENCES

When I was in my baccalaureate program in nursing at Indiana University School of Nursing from 1964 to 1968, I was intrigued that patients who were the same gender, close in age, had similar socio-economic status, and the same disease, at the same stage, could have very different illness experiences. That is, they had quite different pain levels, incidence or intensity of gastrointestinal symptoms (nausea, diarrhea, abdominal cramping, constipation), incidence of fatigue, and insomnia. It was easy to make comparisons at that time because patients were on open wards and assigned to a ward based on gender and disease type. I thought maybe the courses I was taking would help me understand something about the underlying reasons for the different illness experiences I was observing, but I hoped to no avail. Of course, we learned that everyone was different and each patient needed to be understood as a unique person, but that information wasn't any help in understanding what contributed to each person's emotional and physical responses to their hospitalization experiences.

Although I didn't learn what might be underlying the difference in illness experiences in people with the same disease and similar demographics, I did learn from Florence Nightingale's work (which I was studying at the time) that illness and disease are two very different phenomena. Unfortunately, this truth is not commonly acknowledged in the health care community. I should note here that nursing's unique contribution to health care is grounded in this fact. Florence Nightingale, my hero, wrote about the difference in her 1859 book, *Notes on Nursing*. Her book identified the foundation for nursing's unique contribution to patient care that helps relieve suffering and maintains, or improves, functional ability apart from medical care. Nightingale was very clear that disease, trauma, injury, and illness are very different phenomena. I learned from her work, and that of others, that disease is pathology, that is, abnormal tissue or physiology (pathophysiology). It is objective, meaning that it can be seen and measured. Illness, on the other hand, is subjective and captures how a person is feeling physically, emotionally, and functionally. Lots of factors can influence a person's symptoms (physical and mental) as well as their functional ability that have absolutely nothing to do with disease, not the least of which is psychological stress. That insight is what has guided my own study and research to this day.

## THE CAUSES OF STRESS

I knew, while an undergraduate student, that I eventually wanted to teach. In 1969, I enrolled in Indiana University's Master of Science in Nursing program, focused on preparing Clinical Nurse Specialists in Medical-Surgical Nursing with a minor in teaching. One of our required courses focused on Psychosocial Dynamics of Patient Care and introduced me to the work of Richard Lazarus. He was a distinguished scholar, researcher and professor at the University of California, Berkley. As a social psychologist doing research on psychological stress, he published his landmark book, *Psychological Stress and Coping*, in 1966. Lazarus's book incorporated a critical review of the stress research done to date, including research on emotions and results of the many studies that he and his colleagues had conducted. I knew right away that his work would help to explain the different illness experiences I had seen, and continued to see, in patients.

Unfortunately, by the late 1960s, Hans Selye's General Adaptation Syndrome theory of stress, based on his research using rats as subjects, had taken center stage as the explanation of psychological stress in the medical and health care community. Really?! Extrapolating from research findings using rats as subjects to try to explain psychological stress in humans just didn't make sense to me. Complicating matters was the fact that social psychology, including the use of human subjects, was not popular in the 1960s. Additionally, B.F. Skinner's explanation of behavior, based on reward and punishment, was also center stage. The focus on B. F. Skinner's work in the 1960s contributed to a major war between psychologists. On one side were behaviorists, who argued that emotions were triggered externally through reward and punishment, and on the other side were the cognitivists, who had research data on human subjects demonstrating that thoughts triggered emotions. In large part Lazarus's work on stress and coping went unnoticed for quite some time because of this war of ideas.

Lazarus's research was groundbreaking and soon became the focus of my own study because it confirmed something that I was seeing in my practice: that emotions are triggered by a person's appraisal of a situation. That is, thoughts trigger emotions. He asserted that events are not good or bad, but the meaning we give events determines how we feel. He also identified the two conditions necessary for stress to occur: the demands of your situation exceed the resources you have available and you perceive the situation as threatening.

Lazarus's theory of stress and coping based on sound research made a lot of practical sense to me and explained a good deal of why patients had such different illness experiences. Richard Lazarus joined Florence Nightingale in my pantheon of heroes, and I decided that it was stress and stress-related physical illness that I wanted to make my specialty focus.

## LOWERING BLOOD PRESSURE

I graduated with my Master of Science in Nursing (MSN) degree in 1971 and began to teach in the MSN program in the fall of 1971.

Along with two psychiatric Clinical Nurse Specialist faculty members at the school, I developed a course on the Dynamics of Stress and Coping and began teaching it in 1973. The course focused on stress theory and research as well as on stress counseling skills to use with patients. It remains a course offered today in the MSN program.

In 1974, I decided that I wanted to start my own private practice with individuals who were suffering from stress-related physical illness. I didn't know if I would need the skills of a Nurse Practitioner, a role just beginning at that time, so I enrolled in an NP certificate program – there were no master's degrees for that role at the time. It was a nine-month, five-day-a-week intensive program that the school of nursing supported me in attending. It was only after three months in the program that I knew I did not need the medical diagnostic skills to be effective in the private practice I was planning. I completed the program in 1975. During the program's clinical practicums, I was able to confirm that I was going to offer a service that patients needed. Each day, after I met the clinical requirements for the program, both the family practice MD and internist MD allowed me to see patients who might need my services. Their decision to include me in their practices was the most important affirmation I could receive at the time.

In 1976, I started my practice in conjunction with an MD internist who was a faculty member at I.U. School of Medicine. Working in partnership with him gave me access to patients and gave me an opportunity to demonstrate that patients would be willing to pay for the services (the services provided during my time with the internist were gratis). I'll never forget my first patient, who I was able to see before her physician did. She was a CPA returning for a follow-up visit for hypertension. This was in late March, the middle of a heavy corporate tax season. She had been overwhelmed with her workload for three months at the financial firm where she worked. At her appointment one month prior, she was given a working diagnosis of Essential Hypertension and was advised to start a low salt diet and put on diuretics. This was her follow-up visit to see if the low salt diet and diuretic would be sufficient treatment for her elevated blood pressure.

I was able to talk with her for fifteen minutes before the doctor came in. He took her blood pressure, and it was still elevated. He said to her, "I'm going to have to prescribe an antihypertensive medication." I thought to myself, "I really think the elevation is stress-related," so I asked if he would be okay with me taking her through an autogenic relaxation exercise and, then, check her blood pressure again. He agreed, but he wanted to be the one to take her blood pressure. He stayed in the room while I guided her through the exercise that you'll see discussed in Chapter six. When we finished, he took her blood pressure and just said, "Would you be willing to work with Brenda on your stress?" She said yes, and he turned around and tore up the prescription he had written. How fortuitous that my first patient was such a great example of the role stress can play in our physical health! After two months and six visits, that patient was able to learn how to eliminate and prevent stress in difficult situations and keep her blood pressure within normal limits.

## SPREADING THE MESSAGE

Although I had very meaningful experiences helping patients learn how to deal with stress while I was in the Nurse Practitioner program, this experience with my first patient at the medical diagnostic clinic at I.U. had me hooked. I knew I needed to open up a private practice. I rented an office in the Indiana State Nurses Association building and began to see patients who found me by word of mouth. All of my clients who had continuous physical symptoms had to have been seen by an MD to rule out any possible disease-based causes for their physical symptoms.

In 1977, I began my Doctoral studies in Nursing at I.U. My private practice, and the nationwide workshops I conducted on how to prevent and eliminate stress, supported me financially through my doctoral program. I finished the program in 1981 and was given a faculty position as an Associate Professor at the school once again.

In 1982, I co-founded, with Dr. Joan Werner, the Midwest Nursing Research Societies (MNRS) Stress And Coping Research Section. I was honored to chair the planning and research critique team for MNRS's first knowledge synthesis conference, presented in 1992. I chaired the same group for the second knowledge synthesis conference, presented in 1994. We were honored to have Dr. Richard Lazarus attend our conference and to be one of our presenters. He wrote a chapter for the very popular academic book, *Handbook of Stress Coping and Health: Implications for Nursing Research, Theory, and Practice* published in 2000, for which many of us, as members of the research section, wrote chapters. Unfortunately, Dr. Lazarus died too early in 2002 in a tragic accident. He was a great researcher, academician, author, and colleague. His work not only informed my practice, it provided the foundation for my observations and clarifications on the thoughts that trigger each of the stress emotions.

In 1985, I was able to open up the Office for Nursing Practice under the auspices of the School of Nursing with four other faculty whose specialties focused on providing nursing services to patients. It was no small feat to establish this at a medical center where the school of medicine was not happy with nurses independently providing nursing services! The Office of Nursing Practice operated for 15 years at the school until processing clients' payments for services became too complicated, and I was the only faculty member left providing services.

After we closed the Office for Nursing Practice, I saw clients again in a rented office space and, then, later, in my home. I retired from I.U. School of Nursing in 2010 as a Professor Emerita. I continued my private practice until 2014. During my career, in addition to my work with individual clients, I was privileged to conduct over 350 workshops on stress management and conquering stress for corporations, health professional groups, and trade associations.

## GRATITUDE

I am honored to have been inducted, as a Fellow, into the interdisciplinary National Academies of Practice, in 1988, in recognition of my work in the field of stress. I was also inducted as a Fellow into the American Academy of Nursing, in 1993, in recognition of my contributions to nursing as a discipline and my work in the field of stress. In 1995, I received the Midwest Nursing Research Society Stress And Coping Research Section's Outstanding Achievement in the Advancement of Stress & Coping Science Award.

Although the recognitions I have received are nice, it is my private practice, and what I have learned from that work, that is most gratifying to me but perhaps for a reason you may not be able to anticipate. The skills I've learned, to manage my thoughts and process my feelings about my own disease, have helped me keep stress at bay.

I was first diagnosed with stage IIIA lobular breast cancer in 1997. It was shocking because I didn't have a family history of breast cancer and had just had a negative mammogram four months earlier. Soon after hearing the diagnosis, my head went to, *I'm going to die from this!* Of course, that thought triggered anxiety, and I wasn't able to eat or sleep. After a little over a week I said to myself, "Brenda, you know how to stop the anxiety. Just do it." I sat down and wrote, probably thirty times: "This is NOT a death sentence! I can handle this!" I also used the techniques I had taught, like focusing on the present, which I will share in this book. By the evening of that day, the anxiety was gone, and I was able to focus on how I was going to deal with cancer in a positive manner.

It wasn't until 2014 that the cancer came back. It had metastasized to all of my upper body bones. I had no pain, but the cancer in the ribs caused a pleural effusion (fluid between the ribs and the lining of the lung on the left side). Fourteen years! I was so grateful that it took that long to show up again. As of the writing of this book, I'm on my fifth different drug but still going strong almost 23 years after initial diagnosis. I live life everyday feeling well, being grateful and looking forward to my travels and being with family and friends. I share this part of my story with you to let you know I have been there, and I personally know not only what life-altering stress can feel like but also that what I am sharing with you really works.

Before I begin showing you how to take control of your stress, stress emotions, and the negative effects on your health, I want to thank my private clients for all that they helped me learn from treating their stress and stress-related illnesses; I also want to thank you for picking up this book and giving it a try. Together, we'll move forward in the ongoing (and from where I'm sitting, successful) battle to conquer stress!

Enjoy the journey!
Brenda L. Lyon PhD, CNS, RN

# CHAPTER 1

# RETHINKING STRESS

Change your thinking, change your life.

—FRANK SONNENBERG

Every day, on television, in magazines and online, we hear or read about how important it is to take care of ourselves. Most people, when they hear or read this advice, immediately think, Okay, but how *exactly* should I do that? The answer to that question tends to be: increase exercise, meditate, cut out junk food, go on vacation and reduce stress, which is very hard to do when you are stressed. And how can you take control of your stress when you've always been told that it's simply an ever-present fact of life, caused by what is happening around you and to you? Most people have tried all of the recommended stress reduction techniques to no long lasting avail. No matter how much physical activity you get, how many relaxation exercises you do, or how you change your eating habits, you will feel good while you're doing them, and for a short time afterwards, but those remedies never have lasting effects. For most people, it's become increasingly apparent that, when it comes to stress, once that horse is out of the stable there is no getting it back in. Working on managing stress is never a satisfying experience because it simply does not work.

But what if you could prevent stress or truly *eliminate it* when experienced? What if you didn't have to experience the anxiety attacks, agitation, fear, anger, back pain, stomach pain, and all the other unpleasant things that stress brings with it? What if constant stress management, which seems to be an integral part of life, just disappeared? Think of how many things would change. Then think about what effect those changes would have on other aspects of your life. The positive ripple effect could be endless.

Sure, it's a challenge to take charge of your thoughts to prevent stress, and its damaging effects on your life, but you can do it! To get there, you must first understand: 1) why you have not had success managing your stress until now, 2) what causes stress and 3) what is behind all of the ways that you experience it.

Why you haven't been able to eliminate your stress successfully: It isn't you!

The answer to what seems like an unsolvable puzzle is actually pretty simple and straightforward: The most popular strategies recommended to manage stress grew out of research that has been disproved.

Let that sink in for a second.

Most of the articles you've read about stress, managing stress, getting rid of stress, and learning how to talk about your stress are based primarily on one person's research from over sixty years ago that was disproven decades ago. Obviously, it's infuriating that information is being shared with the average person that is not going to help them, and trying them is a waste of precious time. It is also incredibly irritating to realize that we could have been a nation of infinitely more relaxed and effective people, for a very long time, if only we had known the truth. It amazes me that the amount of stress experienced daily by most people really has not improved, much less changed, since I entered the field in the 1970s. In fact, if anything, the amount of stress experienced by most people is higher. This is increasingly expensive, both in terms of economic cost and emotional health.

In this chapter, we're going to explore the most popular outdated strategies to manage stress, where they came from, and why they are ineffective. We're also going to investigate what stress is, signs of stress and the causes of stress that you *can* control. This is based on up-to-date research that has been confirmed by studies and applied to real people in real stress situations. In other words, the good news is that you can both prevent and eliminate stress, so let's begin!

## EVERYTHING YOU THINK IS TRUE ABOUT WHAT CAUSES STRESS IS LIKELY WRONG!

The most popular and promoted strategies to manage stress, such as eating right, exercising, meditating, relaxing emanate from the theory formulated by Hans Selye, MD. Selye was a researcher in Canada who tried to identify hormonal responses to toxic stimuli by studying rats in the laboratory from the 1930s through the 1950s. Although he didn't identify any new *hormonal* responses, Selye did see a pattern in the *physical* changes that occurred in his rats. Regardless of the type of toxic harm (extreme heat, chemical burns, starvation) he applied to the rats, Selye consistently saw anatomical and physiological signs of enlarged adrenal glands, signs of a depressed immune system, and bleeding ulcers in stomachs and intestines. He concluded that what he was seeing was a newly identified phenomenon, which he called stress.

Selye defined stress as a nonspecific response to any type of toxic experience. This means that no matter what kind of stressor an individual had to deal with, the body would always react in the same physiological way, with the same anatomical changes. Selye went on to formulate his theory of General Adaptation Syndrome (GAS), which asserted that you are born with a certain amount of adaptive energy and every time you experience a significant demand, some of your energy store is depleted. To put it more simply, it's like having a bank account that has a fixed amount of money in it, and, every time you withdraw money, you deplete your account until there is a zero balance. If you try to go below your zero balance, you don't have the benefit of overdraft . . . you just die.[1,2,3] Well, now that is a gas!

As if Selye's theory were not already appealing enough, he went on to say that thoughts (or how you perceive a situation) play absolutely *no* role in your body's response to external demands. If you've been alive for more than five minutes, you know that doesn't sound right. The problem is that Selye did his research on rats, who are less inclined than humans are to share the inner workings of their emotional lives. Nonetheless, Selye's GAS theory became the standard, not only for what defined stress, but also for explaining its occurrence. The theory was adopted world-wide and was incorporated into medical and nursing textbooks, and why wouldn't it be? If Selye's theory was correct, it not only had the possibility of curing serious medical issues, it would be essential to teach everyone that the best self-care recommendations to manage stress were to eat right, practice meditation, learn how to relax, exercise and participate in diversional activity. By incorporating these activities into your lifestyle, you would be in a constant state of trying to preserve your energy stores to get ready for the daily onslaught of stress.

Selye's theory, flawed as it is, made perfect sense when he developed it; at that time, there was a severe lack of appreciation of the role the mind plays in human illness experiences. Medical research used only animals for experimental research and the medical model for health care, including diagnosis and treatment, focused only on the pathophysiology of disease. Doing research only on animals (and not on humans) makes sense if thoughts and emotions play no role in illness or disease experiences. Unfortunately, this medical model, which does not consider the effect of a person's thoughts and emotions on illness experiences, is widely accepted today.

## BENEFITS OF SUPPORT ON STRESS

Despite the popularity of Selye's GAS, it just didn't make sense to Dr. John Mason, a research scientist at Walter Reed Hospital. In the 1970s, Mason conducted experiments applying the same stressors to the rats that Selye did but changing the conditions under which the stressors were applied. For example, he changed the environment the rat was in while the stressor was applied, or gradually increased the toxicity of the stressor. In one of his studies rather than applying the stressor to a rat in isolation, the stressor was applied to a rat while in the company of other rats. Although Mason recognized that rats have limited cognitive ability, he knew that rats showed signs of being able to perceive danger. Well, lo and behold the rats in his experiments showed very different responses than those observed by Selye.[4,5,6,7] Mason's rats did not show the anatomical and physiological signs of enlarged adrenal glands, signs of a depressed immune system, or bleeding ulcers in stomachs and intestines that Selye had found. Mason's work really was the first research on the psychological effect of social support on the experience of stress. Mason's results make sense. For me, and probably for you too, it is helpful to have supportive people around in difficult situations.

Mason's research absolutely disproved Selye's theory, which didn't even hold true for rats! Once Mason's findings were published, there was no shortage of people in the field who thought it might be worth a few minutes' time to revisit the incontrovertible results of Selye's research. Unsurprisingly, Selye's GAS theory was criticized for not accounting for the psychological variables in the stress experience.

He responded by writing *"Forty Years of Stress Research: Principal Remaining Problems and Misconceptions."* in 1976. In this article, Selye attempted to incorporate psychological variables that would help to support his theory, in large part by asserting that there was such a thing as eustress or positive stress. Well now, that's really interesting. In *my* forty years in the field I've never had anyone say to me, "Brenda, you wouldn't believe how much stress I'm experiencing and how good it feels!"

## A GAP IN KNOWLEDGE

I had the opportunity to present at a major national conference with Selye and several other stress researchers including Richard Lazarus in 1980. The focus of my presentation was the role of self-talk in creating psychological stress. Selye's research focus was on what outside stressors do to the body, not on the role the mind plays in causing of stress. So, as you can imagine, we had a great conversation. To my surprise and delight, he found my presentation fascinating. When we met, he was the most gentle and well-intentioned physician I had ever met. In his 1976 article, Selye asserted that perception and interpretation of experiences were not included in his theory because such factors were outside his expertise as a physiologist. This seemed an affirmation of the importance of what the mind's eye sees, but that Selye was not able to account for it because of his knowledge limitations. We'll never know. However, it is important to realize that Selye's line of reasoning was entirely in line with main stream medicine, and unfortunately is still common today.

It is amazing that so many recommended strategies to manage stress today grew out of a disproven theory. It reminds me of what a good physician friend said to me years ago, "Brenda the questions in medicine never change much. Only the answers change!" How true!

I learned this lesson the hard way when I was diagnosed with breast cancer after years of the medical community telling us that there was absolutely no correlation between estrogen and breast cancer. In fact, we were told based on research, that estrogen helped protect the heart in females. Then when I was diagnosed in 1997 my surgical oncologist said to me that we have to do further testing on the biopsy to determine if the cancer is estrogen sensitive. I said, "What do you mean? I thought there was no correlation?" Well that research was flawed! Nice to know after being on estrogen for five years to address insomnia caused by menopause. I'm not saying that estrogen was the only factor causing my breast cancer, but with no family history, estrogen had to play a role. What's the moral of the story? Think critically about the science!

It is good that many high school students today are taught the basics of research. We can only hope that, although the level of research knowledge taught in high school is minimal, it's enough to help people think critically about research findings and not to accept them blindly.

## THE LIFE CHANGES EXPLANATION OF STRESS

Another very popular explanation of stress is the Life Event Theory developed during the late 1960s and early 1970s by Thomas Holmes and Richard Rahe at the University of Washington School of Medicine.[9,10] Holmes and Rahe wanted to understand the impact that common life changes had on a person's health. So they developed a survey that listed a large number of common life changes. They first had to determine the amount of adaptive energy each change required. Since both Holmes and Rahe were associated with the Navy they used a convenient large sample of Navy recruits during the Vietnam era. They administered the survey with Navy recruits asking them to imagine on a scale of 0-100 how much adaptive energy each change would take. The amount of energy required was called a Life Change Unit or LCU.

Based on their research with Navy recruits, they created the *Social Readjustment Rating Scale* (SRRS) that eventually contained 43 common life changes each with an assigned number of LCUs. They arrived at a score for each event by calculating the average of the ratings given to it by the Navy recruits. When you take the SRRS survey you are asked to sum up the total LCUs that you have experienced within the last year. Your total score is your total life change score.

Using the SRRS, Holmes and Rahe then conducted research following subjects who had taken it to establish a life change score and then tracked the subjects over a year's time, tracking their illness experiences, including but not limited to colds, doctor visits, medical diagnoses, and hospitalizations. From their research, they concluded that, if a person scored over 300 LCUs on the scale, the individual had an 80% chance of experiencing a physical or mental illness within the next year.[11] Based on the Holmes and Rahe research, the (flawed) conclusion was that the most important stress management strategy was to control how many changes occurred in your life and to keep your life changes to a minimum. Even the evening news media went wild about this research, discussing how important it was to take the SRRS and to keep the number of changes you experience to a minimum. Change and stress came to mean the same thing.

While this was a popular theory, it did not hold up. Hundreds of studies of people over time, examining the relationship between the score on the SRRS and getting sick found that the score on the tool only accounted for only four to six percent of the incidence of illness. That leaves 94-96% of the incidence of illness totally unaccounted for by a person's score on the SRRS. The problem with Holmes and Rahe's research is that relying on the imagination of teenage navy recruits, who haven't experienced many of the changes listed by Holmes and Rahe, to accurately judge how much adaptive energy each one of those changes might require, is a bit problematic, to say the least. In addition there are other problematic assumptions underlying the research conducted by Holmes and Rahe. One of the most problematic is the assumption that all of us experience a particular life change in exactly the same way. Research must take into account what the change means in any particular person's life and whether that person has experienced the change before. Everyone is different and everyone's situation is different, which pretty much discredits Holmes and Rahe's findings. (Their model is, however, interesting, especially if you like crunching numbers.)

## HARDINESS AND STRESS

Before anyone could get too comfortable with Holmes and Rahe's research conclusions, Suzanne Kobasa came along and disproved their theory while studying hardiness.[12,13] Hardiness is the feeling of courage and motivation that occurs when a person is interested in and curious about life, feeling a sense of control and viewing change as an opportunity for growth. Kobasa found that hardiness was a potent factor in determining how an individual experienced life changes. That is, a person who had a strong sense of control, confidence in self, and a positive sense of meaning did not experience negative illness related outcomes from life changes. This makes sense and it's great that Kobasa confirmed what many on the planet already knew. There were many other researchers, such as Irwin Sarason, et al[14] who also disproved the Holmes and Rahe theory.

Despite the fact that The Life Event Theory was disproved by Kobasa and others it remained popular, perhaps because its an easy way to recognize and define stress by just adding up scores on a survey tool. Nonetheless, ease of comprehension doesn't mean that a theory is any good or that it will encourage people to make great life choices. When I did workshops on stress management, there were people in the audience who were at my workshop because they were concerned about their health after taking Holmes and Rahe's SRRS and scoring over 300 points. I even had a private client, who was in a psychologically abusive marriage and really needed to get a divorce, come to me because she was concerned that, if she did leave her husband, she'd develop some dreadful disease (based on her SRRS score). After I assured her that the research findings had been invalidated and that the score was really meaningless, she got the divorce and started a new life disease free.

Fortunately, there is another explanation of the nature of stress that has abundant research support and, frankly, just makes practical sense. That is the work of one Richard Lazarus, a social psychologist who conducted his research in Berkley, California. In the next few sections, we will take a look at Lazarus's theory and other research on the nature of stress.

## WHAT IS STRESS?

Put simply, Richard Lazarus's definition of stress is that it is an uncomfortable emotional experience that occurs when you view a situation as potentially harmful to you, or to something or someone important to you, and the situation requires coping effort on your part.[15] In other words, stress happens when you *think* that something bad is going to happen and you have to deal with it. Lazarus described stress as encompassing your interpretation of a difficult situation, your emotions in the situation and how you cope with the situation. Stress is not an event and cannot be measured as a single experience or event. Lazarus's research studies, and hundreds of other studies, have confirmed or supported his explanation of both stress and coping.[16] In other words Lazarus's explanation of stress holds true for humans! Stress is *not* something that happens to you. It's about what you *think* about what has happened or what is happening. Thanks to Lazarus, we know that difficult situations and stress do not have to go hand in hand. They are not the same thing!

## WHAT DOES STRESS FEEL LIKE?

Prior to the 1980s, the word stress was not a part of our everyday vocabulary to describe how we felt when experiencing difficult circumstances. People typically identified the particular emotion felt when stressed with words like overwhelmed, anxious, nervous, angry, or guilty. Unfortunately, now people tend to say things like, "I'm stressed out" or "You can't believe how much stress I'm experiencing." The difficulty created by using such phrases to describe what you feel is that you can't get your arms around them. They're too general and lack any meaningful descriptors.

Even if you don't know how to define or express stress, generally a person knows when they are stressed because they will experience physical, emotional, and behavioral signs. Common physical signs of stress include, but are not limited to, tension headaches, digestive disturbances, muscle stiffness, hyperventilation, sweating, and fatigue. Common stress emotions are feeling overwhelmed, anxiety, anger, guilt, and frustration. Common behavioral signs of stress are irritability, impatience, angry outbursts, inability to relax, trouble sleeping, no energy for tasks.

## WHAT CAUSES STRESS?

Here's the basic description of what causes stress: Stress occurs when the demands of a situation outweigh the resources you have available to *comfortably* deal with it, and you, in turn, believe that there is potential for some type of harm or loss. This perceived potential for harm or loss is also called, in the theory, perceived threat. Our friend, Dr. Lazarus, identified the causes of stress in 1966. What the situation means to the person, and how significant it is in their lives, determines if the situation is neutral, challenging, or threatening. If the situation is perceived as threatening, then one must determine how to cope with the situation. The bottom line is that stress is experienced when the following two conditions are met:

1. You experience a situation as one in which the *demands* **are greater than the** *resources* **you have** available to comfortably deal with it.

2. You *anticipate* **experiencing some kind of harm/loss or negative outcome** (referred to as a **threat**).[17,18]

## STRESS SIGNALS

### EMOTIONAL SIGNALS

- ☐ Feeling overwhelmed
- ☐ Frequent anxiety
- ☐ Frequent anger
- ☐ Frequent guilt
- ☐ Frequent frustration
- ☐ Feeling down/the blues

### PHYSICAL SIGNALS

- ☐ Tension headaches
- ☐ Digestive disturbances (heart burn, diarrhea, constipation, loss of appetite, increased appetite)
- ☐ Muscle stiffness/tightening
- ☐ Hyperventilation (rapid/ shallow breathing)
- ☐ Sweating
- ☐ Fatigue

### BEHAVIORAL SIGNALS

- ☐ Irritability
- ☐ Impatience
- ☐ Angry outbursts
- ☐ Unable to relax
- ☐ Trouble sleeping
- ☐ No energy for tasks
- ☐ Nail biting
- ☐ Fidgeting

PREREQUISITES FOR STRESS

DEMANDS > RESOURCES

+

ANTICIPATED HARM/LOSS
(THREAT)

## ELIMINATING STRESS

Now here's the good news: Although both conditions are necessary for you to experience stress, **each also presents an opportunity for you to prevent or reduce it**. You can:

- Change the situation by *reducing controllable and non-essential demands* and/or by increasing your resources to meet them.
- *Choose to focus on the potential for gain or benefit in a situation rather than potential harm* . . . even if it's just what you will learn from the situation.

Chapters two through five explore how you can effectively address each of these pre-requisites to both prevent and eliminate stress. Here is a basic overview of a few of the main concepts in those chapters to get you thinking in the right direction.

There are many things you cannot control: the weather, environmental catastrophes, accidents, certain diseases, others' expectations, and the imperfections of others. But there is still hope! Even when you cannot control or change the situation, **you can control or change what you choose to think about it or how you choose to view it.**

For example, yes, it's absolutely awful if your home is destroyed by fire or a tornado, or you're laid off from your job, or you discover that your spouse is having an affair, or you're diagnosed with a life-threatening disease. However, it is how you perceive the event (the meaning you place on it), or what you choose to focus on, while immersed in difficult situations, that determines how you feel! The wonderfully amazing fact is that it is *really your choice*. It's not the thing that happens that creates how you feel, it is *what you choose to think about and focus on in the situation that creates your feelings*. In other words, *you* are in control of you, the situation is *not*. I've worked with clients who were able to frame the destruction of their home as an unplanned opportunity to make long desired design changes, even viewing the transition time as an adventure.

## REFRAMING A PAINFUL SITUATION

A poignant story of reframing a painful situation comes from David, one of the people I've worked with on issues related to stress. David had been married for 26 years to his high school sweetheart. She was his everything, the perfect wife and the perfect mother for 21 of those years. During their 23rd year of marriage, he discovered that she had been having an affair with a good family friend. He was devastated, but she was remorseful and convinced him that she loved him and that it was a *big* mistake for which she was ashamed and sorry. They agreed to work on their relationship and, after three years, everything seemed to be back to normal. David got a new exciting job that paid more with even better benefits. Life was going to be great!!

Then, two weeks after starting his new job, he discovered that his wife's affair never ended and that she wanted a divorce. He was absolutely devastated, even worse than the first time, realizing that his life, as he thought, wasn't real. Stricken with incredible grief and anger, he was not able to function at his new job and considered ending it all because she was his whole life. David's employer was incredibly accommodating to him and encouraged him to seek help, to contact the employee assistance program and to see his physician. David's employer connected him with me. David's physician wanted him to go to a local hospital that had excellent psychiatric and counseling services, both inpatient and outpatient. He was being encouraged to go for inpatient assistance because he was having suicidal thoughts. He refused to go someplace with a lot of crazies! I was able to talk with David over the phone while he was staying at home from work trying to figure out his next move. David shared his story with me while almost uncontrollably crying. "There's nothing for me now…she was everything to me…I've lived my life for her!" I acknowledged David's incredible grief, a deep seated painful hurt and almost unbearable sadness. After about twenty minutes of discussion I had this exchange with David:

> Me: I'm going to ask you a question that will seem absolutely ridiculous, but I want you to think about it and see if you can give me an answer. What's one positive thing about this whole situation? *I waited for at least 2 minutes (it seemed like an eternity).*

> David: I can't think of anything . . . . There's absolutely nothing . . . it's just all awful!!

> Me: Does Jennifer (his wife) have the same positive attributes today as the Jennifer you married? The person that helped raise your children. Is she the same person that you have idealized?

David: Absolutely *NOT* . . . . She's a different person . . .
almost everything about her is different . . . even her
core values.

Me: So, would you want to live with the new Jennifer for the
rest of your life?

David: [After pausing briefly] . . . Actually, *No* . . . I would be
miserable!

Me: So, is it possible that she is doing you a favor by asking
for a divorce . . . as difficult as it is now it means you can
start a new life and not be miserable.

David: You know, you're absolutely right! When you look
at it that way ... I really wasn't happy the last 3 years
because I knew deep down something wasn't right
... it's like I was pretending it was OK. She is actually
doing me a favor!

After another ten minutes of conversation, including assuring
him that the hospital had the people to help him get through this
incredibly devastating situation, he asked for a hospital referral. After seven days of inpatient care, David attended weekly outpatient
group counseling sessions. Incredibly, after six months David became a co-leader volunteering to help with the sessions! He is now
remarried and says that he is happier than he can ever remember.

David isn't alone in this kind of experience. Jane, who holds an
MBA, was devastated when she was suddenly laid off from a well-pay-
ing job where she had influenced the institution's outcomes positively over 15 years. When she met with me, she didn't know where to
start, "Besides being angry, I'm just plain lost, not feeling positive
at all about my future." We started our discussions on how changes
like this, although initially devastating, can actually be a blessing by

opening up new opportunities. Jane began to talk about the fact that, although she really enjoyed her co-workers, she was getting bored and not feeling stimulated in her job. She developed a plan to update her resume and to begin her job search. It took about six months (a good reason to have a six-month emergency fund saved up), and she landed a fabulous job that actually paid 150% of what she was making before. I just ran into her a few months ago at the grocery store, and she said to me, "Brenda, it's been great. I'm continually challenged, and I've already been promoted."

Ultimately, it is your thoughts that trigger your stress. When you are thinking, you are using words. Words have meanings, and you *feel* the positive, negative, or neutral meaning of words. An example would be instead of saying, *"This situation is awful,"* you could instead say, *"Now this is the type of situation that builds character!"* In the first instance, you feel bad and disempowered, whereas, in the second instance, you feel more energized and empowered. Try this little experiment: Look at the word pairs **I can't** versus **I won't**. Focus on them separately, repeating each silently to yourself.

## I CAN'T VERSUS I WON'T

**I won't** feels better than **I can't.** The phrases *feel* different! That is because the phrase, 'I won't', introduces the notion that you have a *choice*. Research in personality social psychology has demonstrated that perceived degree of choice is directly proportional to the perceived degree of control. That is, the more choice you think you have, the more personal control you actually *do* have.[19]

## THOUGHTS AND EMOTIONS

There is a lot more about the power of words later in this book. For now, hold on to the fundamentally important point that learning to prevent stress is to realize that it is your thoughts that trigger your emotions, and different thoughts trigger different emotions.[20] Becoming aware of your thoughts at times can be difficult because thinking is a lot like breathing. We breathe all the time, but, unless you are having an asthma attack, suffering from a pulmonary disease, or in a smoke-filled environment, you usually are unaware that you are breathing. Likewise, we are often unaware of the thoughts that are triggering our stress emotions. In fact, many times, negative thoughts require absolutely no effort to enter our consciousness because they have become habitual ways of thinking.

## VALUES

Remember this. The foundation for your thoughts is built on your **values, beliefs and attitudes.** Rokeach[21,22] defined a **value** as an ideal regarding how you think you should: be, think, feel and behave. A value is a standard that you hold for yourself. An example of a value is the desire to be a good mother or good father. This value is further defined in terms of what it takes to be a good mother, e.g. I assure that my children have three meals/day, I assure that I spend quality time with my children, I assure that my children are kind to others, I assure that my children are safe, and so on.

**Values act as imperatives for action or 'shoulds' – they drive your behavior.** In fact, when we act inconsistently with a personal value, the resulting emotion is guilt. Incredibly, just the thought of doing something inconsistent with a value can trigger anticipatory guilt and a decision not to engage in the behavior. The potential difficulty arising from values is that values are idealistic in nature. That is, don't take into account what's realistic given a person's real-life situation. The end result is that one could very easily assume that you should be able to do or be all that you value at all times. Nope, that can't be done. You are still human!

## BELIEFS

Now that we've discussed values, let's look at what beliefs are. A **belief** is an assumption or conviction that is held to be true or thought to be factual. Beliefs operate like rules, that is, like instructions on how you and the world around you ought to operate. Beliefs generally contain judgments (e.g., "I believe I'm worthy," "I believe I deserve to be happy," "I believe it's critical to recognize what is controllable and what isn't controllable," "I believe if you change what you think, you can change your life," "I believe everything will turn out all right."). These are positive, healthy beliefs.[24] But, there are also irrational beliefs that are false and quite detrimental. Examples include:

- To be worthy I must be perfect in all that I do
- To be worthy I must be *always* be kind and giving
- To be worthy I must *never* make a mistake
- Life should always be fair to those who deserve it
- If I'm good enough I should be able to make you happy
- If I'm worthy/good enough I should be able to control what other people think or do
- How other people respond to me is a reflection of how I should think about myself
- No one will ever misjudge me . . . if I get a negative response from someone it must be my fault

## ATTITUDES

In addition to values and beliefs, we have attitudes. An **attitude** is a way of being. It represents how we typically view situations, for example, looking for the good in all situations or not. It also represents how we typically respond to people, for example, viewing other people as generally unfriendly or hostile or viewing other people as generally trustworthy. Attitudes represent how we usually respond to things, and they are heavily influenced by our beliefs and values.

Values, beliefs, and attitudes play a significant role in our everyday life. Sometimes values and beliefs conflict with each other. For example, my value of putting forth my best effort at work might be thwarted by the belief that my supervisor will always find fault with what I do, regardless. This type of situation might result in an attitude of complacency, which manifests as not putting forth the best effort along with experiencing both guilt and anger.

I've had the opportunity to work with many career women who are married and have children. For many of these women, the primary cause of their stress is holding simultaneously onto the values of being excellent in career work, excellent as a mother, and excellent as a wife all in the same day because of the belief that I should be able to do it all. Yet, such expectations of self are *impossible*! The resulting attitude is negative, making a woman view life as unmanageable and herself as a failure.

Both values and beliefs shape the way we view ourselves and the world around us. Both influence our perceptions, and, because beliefs are thought to be true, we are assured that what we perceive about a situation, or ourselves, is reality. It's important to know that thoughts are not *facts*! It will be important, as you read through the following chapters, to become aware of both your values and your beliefs because they, in a substantial way, determine what you think. That is, the silent conversations you have with yourself, the emotions you feel, and your subsequent behavior. You will have an opportunity to do a value and belief assessment in Chapter two to help you.

## TIPS FOR BEGINNING YOUR JOURNEY IN CONQUERING STRESS

1.  Remember: stress happens when the demands you are experiencing outweigh the resources you have available to comfortably deal with them.

2.  Identify the demands you experience in your life and which ones you can eliminate, which ones you can delegate, and which ones you can delay attention to. (In Chapter three, you will have an opportunity to identify the demands you experience. Until you get through Chapter three, just become more sensitive to what is requiring extra effort in your life.)

3.  Begin to pay attention to the silent conversations you're having with yourself. Pay attention to the words you use in your self-talk.

4.  Remember how you choose to view a difficult situation determines your level of stress. When you focus on anticipating a negative outcome or loss (threat), you will experience some level of stress.

5.  Start identifying by naming the specific stress emotions you experience, such as anxiety, anger, guilt, and frustration.

6.  Raise your awareness of your values and beliefs. Become more sensitive to your values and beliefs. (There are strategies in Chapters two and three to help you do this.)

7. Recognize that relaxation, exercise, meditation and mindfulness are really good strategies to help calm you and feel good while engaged in these activities, but none of them alone will fix the stress that you are experiencing.

## SUMMARY

The most popular strategies recommended to deal with stress, including eating right, exercising, relaxing, and meditating, are based on disproven theories of what causes stress and stress dynamics. Although all of these efforts are good for your health and feel good while doing them, and perhaps for a short time after, none of them prevent or eliminate what's causing the stress.

The real causes of the stress you experience are: 1) The demands of your situation outweigh the resources you have available to comfortably deal with the situation and 2) You interpret the difficult situation as potentially harming you, someone else, or something important to you. In other words, you view it as a threat.

The wonderful thing here is that you have tremendous control over the non-essential demands you experience, and you have full control over how you choose to view a difficult situation. You can now continue on your journey in learning to both prevent and eliminate stress.

Effective strategies to both prevent and eliminate stress focus in two areas: 1) demand management to eliminate non-essential demands and manage essential demands while also increasing your resources and 2) changing how you view difficult situations from a threat to a challenge opportunity. Seeing the glass half full rather than half empty really is helpful.

The next four chapters focus on the basics of fixing the two conditions that cause you to experience stress and will get you started on an effective path to both prevent and eliminate stress.

# CHAPTER 2

# WHEN DEMANDS AND RESOURCES ARE OUT OF BALANCE

All you can change is yourself, but sometimes that changes
everything!

—GARY W. GOLDSTEIN

Now that we've gone through the basics of defining stress (it's more than the feeling that makes you want to get in bed and stay there), we're going to unpack the meaning of stress even more. The first condition that must be present for you to experience stress is that your demands outweigh the resources you have available to comfortably deal with them. Specifically, we're going to define demands and differentiate between essential and non-essential demands.

We will explore how your values and beliefs drive many of the demands you experience and how your resources help you meet the demands you experience. We will learn what it feels like to be in balance and out of balance or overwhelmed.

An important skill to learn in lowering stress is demand management. To do this effectively, you must be clear on the demands you experience. Therefore, in this chapter there is an emphasis on you being clear about your demands and beginning to get in touch with the values and beliefs that drive you. Yes, this can be a little heavy and requires focused effort to identify your demands, and the values and beliefs that underlie them, but it's worth the effort! Also, just for fun, we're also going to explode the myth of work-life balance.

## WHAT IS A DEMAND?

Life can be full of demands. **A demand is *anything* that requires extra effort: extra thinking, feeling or behaving beyond that which comes automatically to you.** It's helpful to divide demands into two categories, essential and non-essential. **Essential demands** are just that, *essential.* These are demands that it would be a mistake to ignore because

### ESSENTIAL DEMANDS

**Externally Generated:** physical dangers, bad weather, child care needs, parent care needs, maintenance tasks of your home/car, and work tasks.

**Self-Generated:** Personal hygiene, therapeutic self-care needs, such as adhering to a special diet and taking medications, and realistic self-expectations.

### NON-ESSENTIAL DEMANDS

**Externally Generated:** interruptions, noise, and unrealistic expectations of others (coming from situations happening around us that we didn't create, and from other people's needs or desires)

**Self-Generated:** unrealistic self-expectations (expecting yourself to be perfect or to be your "ideal," toxic thoughts, expecting yourself to control the uncontrollable, irrational beliefs you would experience negative consequences. There are two kinds of essential demands, external and self-generated. Examples of essential external demands are physical dangers, bad weather, childcare needs, parent-care needs, maintenance tasks of your home/car, and work tasks. Examples of self-generated essential demands are personal hygiene and therapeutic self-care needs, such as adhering to a special diet, taking medications, and maintaining realistic expectations of yourself.

**Non-essential demands** do not have significant negative consequences if unattended, avoided, or ignored. Like essential demands, non-essential demands originate from your external environment or are self-generated. Examples of external non-essential demands are interruptions, noise, and unrealistic expectations of others (situations happening around us that we didn't create and from other people's needs or desires). Examples of self-generated non-essential demands are expecting yourself to be perfect or your ideal, toxic thoughts, expecting yourself to control the uncontrollable, and irrational beliefs.

> **THE DEMANDS YOU CREATE FOR YOURSELF ARE THE MOST TROUBLESOME!**

Interestingly, for most people, it is the self-generated non-essential demands that are the most troublesome. Even when people find themselves immersed in situations stemming from difficult external demands, they find the self-generated demands to be more stressful and, therefore, more harmful. But, here's the good news, the fact that *you* create your self-generated non-essential demands means you are the one in control![1,2]

## WHAT IS A RESOURCE?

A resource is anything you have within you (like emotional strength or compassion) or around you (like money or friends) that help you get through every day. A few more examples of internal resources are your energy level (eat right and get enough sleep/rest), positive self-esteem, realistic self-expectations, realistic expectations of others, rational beliefs, effective coping skills, and a positive/grateful attitude. External resources include: social support (informational, emotional, instrumental/material, and affirmational), material/financial assets, and a pleasant environment that is physically and emotionally safe.

## WHAT DOES A BALANCE BETWEEN DEMANDS AND RESOURCES FEEL LIKE?

Chances are that you already know what it feels like to be in balance. The easiest way to identify it is simply that everything feels calm and good. You're in a state of equilibrium. Nothing is making you feel nervous, on edge, or hypervigilant. When demands and resources are balanced, it is because you have enough internal and external resources to effectively and comfortably handle whatever internal or external demands you are experiencing. Imagine a rubber band just sitting on your desktop. There's no strain. When you put a demand load on the rubber band by stretching, it works fine until the force (load) placed on it becomes too great. Then, you see the band thinning and becoming lighter in color, and, then, with too much of a load, it breaks. We see this same thing if we visualize an old-fashioned set of scales with your meager resources, represented by a feather, one side and, on the other side, a brick, representing your demand overload. It is no surprise when the brick goes crashing down, and the feather floats away and disappears, right?

Maintaining a balance between demands and resources doesn't mean that you should sit back and stop engaging with the world and never stretch your current knowledge and skills. It doesn't mean that you stop learning new information or skills, such as in a classroom or at work, or refuse a new work role or personal role, like being a new mother or father. It just means that you keep an eye on not feeling *overpowered* by the demands and that you believe you can handle the demands without being overly stressed or breaking down. As you grow and develop as a person, your comfort zone expands, but you still have limits.

It's very important to keep in mind that what is tolerable for one person may not be tolerable for another; you can't judge how someone else is maintaining their balance by comparing them to you. Conversely, you can't judge yourself against other people. Everybody's tolerable demand load is different. For example, imagine that you are a chair. All chairs have four legs or solid base, a seat, and a back. But chairs are made of different materials with different load tolerances and have different designs that affect, not only load tolerance, but also stability. A three-legged chair isn't going to hold up to strain the way a leather wing chair will, right? You're the best judge of what you can and cannot handle because you know yourself better than anybody.

## WHAT DOES AN IMBALANCE BETWEEN DEMANDS AND RESOURCES FEEL LIKE?

When demands substantially outweigh resources, the result is a feeling often described as being **overwhelmed.** You feel frozen, stuck in place, and it's difficult, if not impossible, to take meaningful action to address the situation. Feeling overwhelmed is commonly accompanied by one or more stress emotions, anxiety, anger, guilt or frustration, all of which we'll take a closer look at in later chapters.

It's important to remember that when you describe your feelings (e.g., happy, sad, overwhelmed or in control), words matter. Words carry emotional baggage that can get in the way of whatever situation you're trying to deal with. For example, when you use the word overwhelmed to capture what you're feeling, just saying that word makes the situation *not* manageable! How can you manage feeling overwhelmed when the definition of the word is something that is or feels unmanageable? It's a defeating, downtrodden word. Using that word gives the situation power over you.

If you replace the word overwhelmed with the word **overloaded** in your self-talk your perspective and sense of control changes. Try it out. Say to yourself, I'm overwhelmed! Now say I'm **overloaded.** Does it feel less like you're being taken over by an emotion and more like a description of a practical situation? Dealing effectively with feeling overwhelmed is very difficult, if not impossible, whereas, dealing logically with a practical situation is much more straight-forward. When you frame yourself or your situation as being over-loaded, it reminds you that you're in control and also reinforces that fact. The word overloaded clearly identifies that you need to go into **demand management mode** (reduce non-essential demands and/or increase resources). There are multiple ways to reduce non-essential demands, which you'll learn more about in Chapter three, and just as many ways to increase resources, which you'll find in Chapter four.

## WHAT IS DEMAND MANAGEMENT MODE?

The primary question to ask yourself when feeling overloaded is, **what demands can I unload or eliminate, and what resources can I increase?** Going into demand management mode begins with this question. You're asking yourself how you're going to balance those scales and give the feather some heft to work against that brick. Of course, no one is going to want to let go of or ignore *essential demands*, that is, those demands that are critically important to your well-being and the well-being of those you care about. But before you say, "Yeah, yeah, I know what my essential demands are," and start running through the list in your head that keeps you up at night, consider what your best friend or favorite family member would say about that list. Sometimes, it's helpful to get feedback from others to help in determining the genuine necessity of a demand. It's not uncommon for a person to overestimate the importance of any number of particular external or internal demands.

For example, if you're a parent, is it really critical that you clean your kitchen floor every night for your one-year-old? Unless something really outrageous or gruesome happens in your kitchen on a daily basis, the logical answer is probably no. (For those of you who just shouted, "That's what you think!", research has demonstrated that you can actually be *too* clean and fail to stimulate your child's immune system and prevent it from fully developing at an early age, so there's that.) What if you feel obliged to fully decorate your house for every holiday so your family won't miss out on whatever the seasonal cheer might be? Maybe your family doesn't care as much as you think they do, or, perhaps, they'd help to come up with less arduous ways to celebrate together *if you talk to them about it*. Remember, there are limits to the loads we as human beings can carry, just like those weight limits for chairs we considered earlier in the chapter. In Chapter three, you'll work on identifying the non-essential demands in your life that you generate and have the sole power to eliminate.

As briefly discussed in Chapter one, your values and beliefs are powerful drivers of your self-generated demands. They drive your expectations of yourself, your behavior, and your expectations of others.

1. **Values are standards that represent your ideals or 'shoulds'.**
   Some commonly shared values are *honesty, working hard,* and *kindness.* Other values are organized around the various roles that we have in life, such as being a *good mother,* being a *good wife,* and *being excellent in our job* (**defined differently by each person**). It is helpful to become aware of your values by completing the statement: I desire to be _____, or I should be _____. Then, identify what being _____ looks like in terms of how you think, feel, and behave. We are naturally driven to behave, think, and feel in alignment with our values.

2. **Beliefs are ideas that are assumed to be true or factual.**
   Examples of *positive beliefs* are the following. Everyone I meet is a potential friend. Everything will turn out all right. It's always ok to ask. And, it's always ok to say no. Examples of *irrational beliefs* are the following. Life is always fair to good people. It's not ok to say no. If I take care of others before myself, it will pay off. Loving my husband means that I must accept whatever he does or says. And, If I'm a good enough person, I ought to be able to control how others act and feel.

A particularly problematic belief is the **illusion of control.** When you believe that you can or should be able to control others, you are guaranteed to be disappointed. In fact, when you keep trying to control others, but fail, it invariably feeds a low self-esteem and often leads to situational depression.

Below is a demand/resource assessment that includes common types of non-essential demands and the flip side of these demands as resources. Take a few minutes to put check marks by your current demands and resources.

## MY DEMAND/RESOURCE ASSESSMENT

All of the items discussed below can be <u>DEMANDS</u> (require extra effort, time, feeling, etc.) or <u>RESOURCES</u> (source of support or help to cancel out or meet demands). *IT ALL DEPENDS ON YOUR APPROACH!*

| PERSON SOURCE | DEMAND | RESOURCES |
|---|---|---|
| 1. Your Values - How you desire to be | ☐ Wanting or expecting myself to be perfect<br>☐ Expecting myself to be ideal in situations that are not ideal<br>☐ Needing to be busy to feel valued | ☐ Accepting my imperfections<br>☐ Holding realistic expectations of myself<br>☐ Allowing myself time to recharge |
| 2. Your Beliefs | ☐ Being pessimistic<br>☐ Believing that I should be able to control others<br>☐ Holding onto irrational rules (wanting things done a certain way even if the results don't really matter or are the same for different ways) | ☐ Being optimistic<br>☐ Accepting that I cannot control others<br>☐ Not relying on irrational rules |
| 3. Your Goals | ☐ Setting unrealistic goals (not giving myself enough time to complete tasks)<br>☐ Not breaking large goals down into accomplishable steps | ☐ Setting realistic goals<br>☐ Breaking large goals down into accomplishable steps |
| 4. Your Typical Point of View in Situations | ☐ Viewing situations without humor<br>☐ Focusing on the negative<br>☐ Anticipating the worst | ☐ Viewing situations with humor<br>☐ Focusing on the positive<br>☐ Anticipating the best |

| PERSON SOURCE | DEMAND | RESOURCES |
|---|---|---|
| 5. Your Thought Patterns | ☐ Automatic thinking (assuming that I can read others' minds—what they're thinking)<br><br>☐ Polarized thinking (viewing situations as bad or good, black or white – no grey area)<br><br>☐ Catastrophizing (focusing on the worst possible outcome)<br><br>☐ Blaming others for what I experience<br><br>☐ Should-ing (expecting myself to measure up to my ideal self) | ☐ Not assuming others' motives<br><br>☐ Not thinking in terms of absolutes<br><br>☐ Not thinking the worst of a situation<br><br>☐ Not fixing blame for my difficulties onto others<br><br>☐ Being realistic about what I can do in the situation |
| 6. Your Expectations | ☐ Holding unrealistic expectations of others<br><br>☐ Not being clear about my expectations with others | ☐ Having realistic expectations of others<br><br>☐ Communicating your expectations clearly |
| 7. Your Social Support System | ☐ Isolating myself from others<br><br>☐ Not accepting help from others | ☐ Building relationships with others<br><br>☐ Accepting help from others |
| 8. Your Self-Talk (self-esteem) | ☐ Negative self-talk (talking negatively to myself) | ☐ Positive self-talk |
| 9. Your Coping Skills | ☐ Use emotion-focused, passive strategies | ☐ Use direct action, problem-focused strategies |

| PERSON SOURCE | DEMAND | RESOURCES |
|---|---|---|
| 10. Your Time Management | ☐ Procrastinating<br>☐ Not prioritizing tasks<br>☐ Relying on memory | ☐ Getting tasks done on time<br>☐ Prioritizing tasks<br>☐ Using To Do Lists |
| 11. Your Planning Activities | ☐ Not planning | ☐ Planning |
| 12. Your Diversions | ☐ Not allowing yourself diversions/relaxation time | ☐ Allowing yourself diversions/relaxation time |

**How many demands did you check?** ___

**Think about the last time you experienced stress . . . think about what was happening and what stress emotion(s) you were experiencing. (Identify below.)** _____

_____

_____

_____

_____

**Which of the self-generated demands were operating in that situation? (List)** _____

_____

_____

_____

_____

*EACH NON-ESSENTIAL DEMAND you allow yourself to experience in day-to-day situations increases the likelihood that you will experience stress.*

Now that you've completed your self-assessment, I hope that you are more aware of the non-essential demands that you self-generate and that can be eliminated. Remind yourself that you're the Chairperson of your Board of Directors, and you can choose to go into demand management mode!

## THE MYTH OF BEING ABLE TO DO IT ALL

What does it really look like to be overloaded and eliminate non-essential demands (i.e., go into **demand management mode**)? Let me share an example. Many years ago, a colleague of mine was married to a corporate attorney and had three children ages, eight, 10, and 12. She was working full-time as a faculty member with me and one day said, "Brenda, I'm stressed out. I'm skating on the edge of burning out! Can we go to lunch?" Of course!

During our lunch I asked her what was going on and she said, "The bottom line is I have too much to do. I'm just overwhelmed, and I'm only getting five hours of sleep a night. I'm worn out." I didn't doubt it. She looked distraught and exhausted. I steered the conversation to the topic of demands and how common it is to get caught in an overload mode. I asked her to tell me about all of the demands she was experiencing. My colleague replied, "I work an average of fifty hours per week. I do all the cooking, dishes, laundry, and house cleaning. I help the children with their homework. I usually drive the children to their sports activities, including practices, which are frequent! I sing in the church choir, which requires going to practice. I host dinners for my husband's clients." She wasn't finished. When she stopped to draw a breath I said, "Whoa! that's really a lot. So, what drives you to do everything?" She responded with, "Well that's my job as a mother and wife."

Really? Is it? Her belief that she should do everything imaginable in her domestic life to fulfill her roles as mother and wife, in addition to her faculty role, was driving her over the edge. But, was it really just her belief that she was supposed to do all those things that was driving her, or was it something else? The truth was that what was driving her was her *experience of anticipatory guilt* (a very powerful emotion). She was feeling guilty about a perceived failure *that hadn't even happened yet* that she believed would occur if she didn't meet all of what she defined as her own role expectations. A simple way of putting this is that she was feeling bad because she might, in the future, feel like a failure (by her own measure). Sounds a little out of whack when you think about it that way, right?

My colleague and I went on to talk about how values and beliefs drive expectations of ourselves. Then, we discussed how her role-related values (ideals) and the irrational belief that if she didn't do it all she was a failure was doing her harm. At that moment, it was important that she see that what she was expecting of herself was not humanly possible to do without jeopardizing her own health. I showed her how to make a chart to identify the non-essential demands she was experiencing, the values and beliefs that were driving her unrealistic internal demands, and what to do to eliminate the non-essential demand.

During our second lunch, a couple of weeks later, she showed me her worksheet, including her list of demands and tasks, identifying which ones were essential that she must do and which ones were non-essential (see below). She and her family members sat down together and talked about how the demand load could be shared. Some of the solutions they came up with: She would hire someone to clean her house every other week, she and the children would cook meals to freeze for later, the children would do dishes, and they would even learn to do their own laundry. In addition, her husband was going to drive the children to some practices and games; they would also carpool with parents of other team members. My colleague said, "I feel so much better. I'm already sleeping more, and maybe the best thing is that our children will be learning important life skills." I replied, "Yes, that's true, and you learned an important 'demand management' skill!"

Below is a partial example of my colleague's completed worksheet, including her non-essential demands, the values and beliefs driving those demands, and the fix strategies. After re-reading the overview of values and beliefs, including the illusion of control, that follows my colleague's worksheet example, draw up your own worksheet to fill in.

| SELF-GENERATED Demands, Values, Beliefs & FIX Strategies Worksheet | | | |
|---|---|---|---|
| Non-Essential DEMAND | VALUES (How you desire to be) | BELIEFS (What you think is TRUE) | FIX STRATEGIES |
| Expect myself to be an ideal mother (unrealistic) | Being an ideal mother means I should be able to do everything for my children. | Any mother worth her salt would always put her children first. My children will love me more if I always put them first (e.g., help them with homework and projects, be their taxi driver, go to all activities). | 1. Remind myself that being all of my ideal every day is humanly impossible. 2. Ask myself what I can comfortably accomplish each day. 3. Remind myself that it is not beneficial for children for me to do everything for them. 4. Remind myself that it is critically important that I take care of myself. |

| SELF-GENERATED Demands, Values, Beliefs & FIX Strategies Worksheet | | | |
|---|---|---|---|
| Expect myself to be an ideal wife (unrealistic) | I should be able to be an ideal wife, meaning: I should be able to meet my husband's needs. I should be able to help him be successful (e.g., host client parties, allow him to work quietly at home in the evening, be ok with him playing golf on the weekends). I should clean the house every week and keep things straight. | I will continue to be loved and have a good relationship with my husband if I'm a good (ideal) wife, meaning that everything at home is relatively easy for him. I am the person primarily responsible for the home being managed well. | 1. Remind myself that being all of my ideal every day is humanly impossible. 2. Remind myself that I'm not responsible for my husband's happiness or ease with meeting demands of his career (discuss getting a sitter and going out to dinner with clients, getting a person to come in every other week to clean house). 3. Remind myself that my husband's love for me is not based on the traditional role of wife. |

## FEELING WHAT YOU THINK

Kathryn is another great example of what happens when your demands and resources are out of sync. She came to see me because she was experiencing chronic stomach upset, lost appetite and guilt, along with really low self-esteem. Usually a high performer at work, Kathryn couldn't concentrate as usual and just wanted to do nothing. She had seen her primary care physician, who referred her to a gastroenterologist, after having her try over-the-counter antacids and having blood work done. After all the test results came back as normal, she decided, while talking with a friend, that perhaps it was stress causing her symptoms.

Kathryn was used to feeling like she was in control of everything. She was 37 years old and had established herself as a successful research scientist at a pharmaceutical company. She got married when she was 34. Prior to her marriage, she was able to control her living environment and most of her work environment as she was in charge of her own lab.

After getting married to a man she was truly in love with, a man who was also very successful at work, Kathryn began experiencing chronic anger. She felt her husband was not meeting many of her expectations regarding neatness and organization. After two years of marriage, she started doubting herself because he was showing signs of not being happy. Kathryn thought that was something she should be able to control. After all, she had been able to control everything else. She'd ask over and over, "Why can't I manage him. Why can't I make him happy? There must be something wrong with me."

It didn't take long for Kathryn to learn about unrealistic expectations, chronic anger, and unjustified guilt as well as how to communicate with her husband effectively when expectations weren't met (Chapter eight). She also was able to eliminate her belief that she should be able to control other people and how they feel and, thus, was able to eliminate her unjustified guilt (Chapter seven). That is, each person is responsible for their own emotions and their own behavior.

Once Kathryn started communicating with her husband more effectively and stopped feeling like she was responsible for his happiness, their relationship improved dramatically. She said in her last appointment, "It's really hard to imagine that I didn't learn these things at an earlier age, but I'm grateful to have learned them now!"

Kathryn's story is a perfect example of how your body feels what you think. When you have negative thoughts, your sense of self is negative. If, when you feel that way, you pay attention to how your body feels, you'll notice that you feel less energy or even uncomfortable physical sensations and negative emotions, such as unjustified guilt. Negative self-talk such as, *I should be a better person, I should be stronger, I should be better at what I do*, triggers unjustified guilt. Feeling guilty over time can also contribute to feeling down or experiencing situational depression. When you are able to change how you talk to yourself (your internal dialogue), you'll feel better. We'll get into exactly how you can switch up what you do or don't say to yourself in Chapter three.

## IRRATIONAL BELIEFS

Irrational beliefs give rise to **irrational rules**. Some common irrational rules could be: all the coats in the closet need to hang in the same direction, there's only one way to load the dishwasher, there's only way to run the sweeper, there's only one way to organize the tools in the garage, or there's only one correct way to squeeze a toothpaste tube. It's my way or the highway!

Take some time to make your own worksheet for an assessment of your non-essential self-generated demands, their underlying values and beliefs, and some strategies for fixing or eliminating the demand. You will probably want to revisit your Demand/Resource Assessment to be sure to include the demands you checked there. Additionally, I've given you an example above that should help you in completing your own assessment. You will likely want to revisit this assessment as you progress throughout the book, so I would suggest that you complete your assessment in pencil to allow for erasing, and give yourself plenty of rows to write in.

| SELF-GENERATED Demands, Values, Beliefs & Fix Strategies Worksheet | | | |
|---|---|---|---|
| Non-Essential DEMAND | VALUES (How you desire to be) | BELIEFS (What you think is TRUE) | FIX STRATEGIES |
| | | | |
| | | | |
| | | | |

# WORK/LIFE BALANCE IS A MYTH!

While we're focusing on demands and resources being out of balance, it's worth taking a little time to address the popular but entirely mythical work/life balance idea. Have you ever said to yourself, *I need a better work/life balance*? If you have said that, it means you are experiencing an imbalance in how you want to spend your time. More simply put, you feel that something is being neglected.

The underlying fallacy with the notion of work/life balance is that work and life are binary, meaning that your work life and your home/personal life are totally separate. Not true! Your work life and your personal life are *integrated*. How you think, the demands you experience, the resources you have, and your emotions cut across your work life and your personal life. The question is not: How can I achieve a work/life balance? That question implies that it's a balance of how you spend your time. Balance is not about better time management skills (although that's a good skill). It's rather about balancing your choices of what essential demands you will address and how those demands will be addressed both at work and in your personal life. Instead the question is: How can I focus on only the essential demands in the time I have to achieve a satisfying work life and personal life? We'll answer this question shortly, after considering how the myth got started in the first place.

How did the myth get started that you can reach some magical point in your self-development where all the different demands on you are in sync and you can effortlessly keep everything aloft? The phrase came into use in the late 1980s and early 1990s when there was a huge surge of women entering the workforce. It was important to women to try to find a way to be a good wife, mother, and paid employee all in the same week.

During the 2000s, the new phrase was smart work and applicable across genders. Roughly eighty million millennials entered the workforce with laptops and smartphones, and it was important for businesses to find a way to keep these young workers engaged. The concept of smart work was that you could work anywhere, anytime. An interesting note here is that rather than making it easier to work, it just increased the demand load. Then in 2008 and 2009, with the great recession and the loss of 8.4 million jobs, the new phrase was: Work smart, do more with less. Well that didn't work out well. Employees got angry and burned out. Since 2010, we've returned to work/life balance as the ultimate goal. There are hundreds of articles suggesting how you might achieve that utopian ideal. Despite all that effort, the Occupational and Safety Health Administration (OSHA) estimates that businesses lose $300 billion/year due to stress.

Again, the important question is not, *how can I achieve a work/life balance?* But, rather, *how can I focus on only the essential demands in the time I have to achieve a satisfying work life and personal life?* Remember, essential demands are external (e.g., work life or parent care life), and internal demands (e.g., recharging your batteries, your medical therapeutic care) are demands that, if not met, you would experience some kind of harm or negative consequence. It makes sense to spend some time identifying what your essential demands are and identifying which ones can be delayed or delegated. It's not uncommon to get caught up in the "it must be done today" mode when delaying a day or a few more days or even a week will work. Think about this. Many people have trouble delegating because it's difficult to give up control. More often than not, a task can be completed adequately in many different ways. The outcome is the same, but the method might be different. Think about *that*. To examine how your delegating and organization skills are (or are not) helping you, make and fill in a self-assessment worksheet like the one below. In addition to identifying which demands can be delayed or delegated, identify the priority ranking of each demand. A number one ranking is very important and more urgent than others. A number two ranking represents an important demand but less potential negative consequence if not done in a short time.

## ESSENTIAL DEMAND WORKSHEET

| ESSENTIAL DEMAND | CAN BE DELAYED | CAN BE DELEGATED | PRIORITY RANKING |
|---|---|---|---|
|  |  |  |  |
|  |  |  |  |
|  |  |  |  |

If you're not experiencing satisfaction in your work and personal life, because you're attempting to deal with too many demands, **it really is worth it** to spend some time evaluating your current demands! *It is amazing how many things, if not done, really don't end up mattering very much in terms of negative consequences.* It's also important to identify what is really important. During an intense period at work that requires fifty to sixty or more hours a week of your time, maybe it's more important to spend a few quality hours with your children once a week than it is to spend non-quality time with them every day.

## MANAGING A TEMPORARY SITUATION

Mark is a 32-year-old Project Engineer working for a large manufacturing company. He has held this position for almost a year. He is two months into a six-month project that is requiring that he spend at least 70 hours of work on the project. He leaves home at 7:00 a.m. and gets home at 7:00 p.m. After driving one hour each way, he is exhausted. He often has lunch while he's working. He also has to work a few hours on the weekends. Successful completion of the project is critical to the company meeting its projected financial goals for the year and stockholder expectation. Mark is the only Project Engineer working in his division with the particular skill set required for the project, so he really can't delegate tasks to others. Mark had been used to getting home at 5:30 p.m. and helping with the children, aged seven and nine, with their homework while his wife, a full-time accountant, made dinner. He also played with the children for at least an hour before bed and read them a bedtime story. By the time he gets home and eats, he really has very little time with the children except to read them a bedtime story.

Mark felt trapped in an unending, impossible situation, only fueling his anger that this was not what he expected in the job. He loved his work, but he didn't want to spend the rest of his life working 70 hours a week. Mark was in the forever trap, that is, feeling like the situation you're in has no ending. In fact, Mark's situation at the time was not typical for his job. It's just that the particularly unusual project he was on required his unique skills. Once Mark was able to focus on the fact that the project was limited to four more months of work, he could see the light at the end of the tunnel. He also changed how he viewed the situation from horrible to challenging. He was able to let go of his anger and just roll with it. His wife helped the children with their homework. He talked with the children about not spending much time with them in the evening but, instead, having special times on the weekend. He was able to focus on spending special quality times with his children and his wife on the weekend. He made sure that, during those hours, they got his full attention. It wasn't ideal, but it was satisfying for all.

## TIPS FOR BECOMING AWARE OF WHY YOUR DEMANDS ARE OUTWEIGHING YOUR RESOURCES

1. Pay attention to your demand load! When you feel like demands are getting out of hand, identify those demands that are non-essential and eliminate them. For those demands that are essential, ask yourself which ones can be delegated or delayed.

2. Take care of yourself through nurturing your self-esteem, being careful to be realistic with your expectations of both yourself and others and maintain a grateful attitude. There is more to help you with attending to your internal and external resources in Chapter four.

3. Pay attention to the words you're using in your self-talk. Be careful not to frame a situation where the demands you're experiencing are outweighing your resources as an overwhelming situation. Instead, frame it as an overloaded situation, which triggers my need to go into demand management mode.

## SUMMARY

In this chapter we, 1) defined demands and resources, 2) presented an overview of the types of demands and resources commonly experienced, 3) discussed what balance and imbalance feels like, 4) identified the importance of using language like being overloaded instead of overwhelmed. These internally-generated, non-essential demands increase your demand load and can create an uncomfortable imbalance between what you think you have to do or attend to and the resources you have available to deal with the demands. We also identified some of the values and beliefs that drive the non-essential demands that you self-generate. Hopefully, at this point, you have a sense of what you need to do in a demand management mode to take better care of yourself. Additionally, you've started to think about how to better manage the essential demands in your life so as not be overwhelmed. Also, remember the work/life balance concept is a myth. Don't fall for it!

In Chapter three, we take a very close look at three common non-essential demands: perfectionism, toxic thoughts, and irrational rules. These non-essential demands are particularly challenging to eliminate and, therefore, require some extra time and focus. Chapter three will help you learn how to eliminate these non-essential demands. Although challenging, it's quite doable! Chapter four focuses on strategies to maximize your resources.

Be patient with yourself. Remind yourself that Rome wasn't built in a day, and of the old adage "the only way to eat an elephant is one bite at a time". You *will* make progress in learning how to both prevent and eliminate stress! It is a journey, learning all the way.

# CHAPTER 3

# ELIMINATING NON-ESSENTIAL DEMANDS

*I now realize that instead of saying that I want to 'grow' into my best self, I should say I want to 'reduce' into my best self.*

— KAREN SALMANSOHN

Congratulations! At this point, you have a good understanding of the conditions that must be present for you to experience stress. Now, it's time to learn how to achieve a better balance between demands and resources by eliminating non-essential demands. Learning to do this can go a long way in learning how to prevent stress in the first place. This chapter covers eliminating both self-generated non-essential demands and external non-essential demands.

Let's do a quick review. Remember, a demand is *anything* that requires extra effort on your part. In other words, a demand is not an automatic behavior but, rather, requires your attention and effort. It's like the difference between brushing your teeth on a normal day and trying to brush your teeth if you have a cast on your dominant arm.

Our focus in this chapter is on eliminating non-essential demands. **Non-essential demands** are superfluous, deeply unpleasant, often soul crushing. It is within your power to get rid of self-generated non-essential demands and often within your control to eliminate external non-essential demands. The most common self-generated non-essential demands emanate from: expecting perfection in *any* situation, toxic thoughts (negative situational dialogue and negative self-talk), and behaving based on irrational rules.

I used this analogy in the previous chapter, but it bears repeating! When considering whether or not you can manage the pile of mounting demands in your life, think of yourself as a chair. Just like a chair has a weight, or load, limit that it can handle without breaking, you also have a demand-load limit. In the same way that you know not to put a set of 350-pound barbells on a folding chair, you shouldn't consider putting huge numbers of non-essential demands on yourself; but you do. It's all too common for people to overload themselves! And, when you do, like the folding chair, you'll fall apart.

Now, it's time for you to learn how to rid yourself of the most common non-essential demands and bid that huge unnecessary load you've been carrying around a not-so-fond adieu. Let's get right into it!

## ELIMINATING SELF-GENERATED NON-ESSENTIAL DEMANDS

I'm hoping that you're on board with me now about eliminating non-essential demands from your life. Let's explore how to do that. A word of caution in setting expectations for yourself: Self-generated non-essential demands tend to be troublesome. They are difficult to eliminate because they are well-learned, and they are grounded in your values and beliefs. The good news is that *you* are in control of the demands that you generate. It is *your choice* to continue them or work to eliminate them. As you read through this chapter, and the remaining chapters, continue to reflect on what values and beliefs underlie your self-generated demands. Understanding what your values and beliefs are, and whether they are in sync with how you want to live your life, is an important part of taking control of your stress.

Let's revisit beliefs here. While your personal beliefs are specific to you and your experience, we all have beliefs about ourselves and about the world around us. Those beliefs dictate how we assess the world around us and, also, how we address challenges. Your beliefs can be about anything: your worth, purpose, abilities, your assessment of other people's intentions and fairness. Your beliefs can even be based on the very notions of

> **PERFECTIONISM IS THE BELIEF THAT MISTAKES CAN NEVER BE MADE, AND WE SHOULD ALWAYS MEET THE HIGHEST STANDARD OF PERFORMANCE.**

friendship and love. There are also spiritual beliefs and faith (like the purpose of life and relationships, the potential nature of a supreme being, the existence or nonexistence of an afterlife). Beliefs aren't formed overnight! They are acquired over time, but they can be confirmed, modified, or disconfirmed through experiences. While our instinct is to exclusively regard our beliefs as a source of strength, they can also be a source of problematic demands. The easiest way to identify beliefs that lead to problematic demands is to catch yourself saying "should statements" to yourself. Here are a few examples of problematic beliefs:

- I should (must) be perfect in all that I do so I can be worthy.
- I should feel badly about myself because I am not capable or worthy.

- I should be able to control others' behaviors/feelings.
- If I want something done right, I should (must) do it myself.

These statements sound pretty punishing, right? Would you say any of these to a friend or loved one? Probably not, but we say nasty things like this (or exactly this) to ourselves all the time. We say them so frequently that we may not notice that we do it. However, just because we do not notice what we are doing, it does not mean they have less negative impact on us when we say them. The beliefs listed above create three common internal demands that will inevitably lead to seriously problematic demands or mindsets. These are **perfectionism**, **toxic thoughts** (negative/toxic self-talk) and making decisions based on **irrational rules**. An explanation of each of these demands, and some suggested strategies to eliminate them, follow.

## IDENTIFYING PERFECTIONISM

**Being a perfectionist** generates an almost infinite number of problematic internal demands. As a perfectionist, you might expect your performance to be perfect or ideal in *all* situations. When you set an unattainable goal for yourself, you'll inevitably fall short, causing you to question your coping ability, promoting thinking in absolutes (everything is black or white, never allowing for gray areas), and reinforcing negative self-talk. Don't confuse being a perfectionist with achievement! It's vital to remember that perfection is, by its nature, unattainable. Reasonable high standards may or may not be met, but they don't require you to have superhuman abilities. A perfectionist will commonly perceive a task done as 100% flawless (a very rare occurrence) or 100% failure. A high achiever, however, sets high goals and works very hard to achieve them - if 90% of the goal is achieved, after putting forth a best effort, then it's still satisfying. If 60% of today's to do list is accomplished during a hectic day, with a couple of unexpected interruptions, the accomplishment still feels good!

The perfectionist's negative self-talk creates low self-esteem. But no one is safe. The perfectionist's judgmental eye is not only unfairly critical of self but also critical of others. High achievers, on the other hand, recognize areas for growth and talk positively to themselves about realizing potential. High achievers are also nurturing and supportive of others and view failure as an opportunity to learn something, to improve upon themselves. Typically, high achievers feel good about themselves and have high self-esteem.

> Perfection is NOT a healthy pursuit of excellence.
>
> — UNKNOWN

> I am careful not to confuse excellence with perfection. Excellence, I can reach for, perfection is God's business.
>
> — MICHAEL J. FOX

To understand your own perfectionist tendencies, start with understanding what motivates you to do what you do and behave as you do. Perfectionists are more commonly *motivated by fear* rather than by challenge. *Perfectionists anticipate failure* with any new situation or opportunity that arises, which often triggers an overpowering *fear of failure*. That fear of failure commonly results in chronic dysfunctional anxiety, which makes perfectionists hesitant to take action toward a goal and become immobilized (in other words, paralyzed by fear and worry). Hesitation and paralysis lead to a self-fulfilling prophecy of failure. If you're a writer and frequently experience writer's block, or chronically procrastinate, guess what? You're very likely a perfectionist.[1]

On the other hand, high achievers are able to set priorities and delay attention to some tasks when others take priority. This technique of putting off less important tasks to address vital ones is called functional delay, and it's the one of the biggest weapons in the high achiever's arsenal. For the high achiever, the 40% of tasks that didn't get done today aren't a source of anguish. They are simply rolled over to tomorrow's to do list. A high achiever might prioritize the to do list by assigning importance to tasks by categorizing them as being of A, B or C-level importance. It's likely that the roll-over 40% would be classified as C tasks anyway, that is, nice-to-do tasks but not essential A tasks.

## FUNCTIONAL DELAY

Here's an explanation of **functional delay**. When we have a task that is an A task (really needs to be done) but it doesn't need to be done *right away* (you may have two days, two weeks, or even a month), it's often hard to focus your attention because there is little time pressure to get the task done. In my workshops, I'll ask, "How many of you think you're a procrastinator?" Most people raise their hands. When I say, "Put your hand down if you get an important task done in time even though you may have delayed attending to the task," literally everyone puts their hand down. I coined this phrase "functional delay" because, in fact, it often works very well. I often say that cleaning out a dresser drawer can be a more attractive option than trying to focus on something I must do days in advance.

Of course, sometimes you're motivated to accomplish tasks immediately. But, often, you're easily distracted by some other activity. By putting an unurgent A task off for a little while, you're implementing functional delay, which **creates, or increases, time pressure and, as a result, enhances your ability to concentrate on the task in time for your deadline.** The reality is, unless you are a true procrastinator you will always get your A tasks done on time. Unfortunately, true procrastinators suffer the consequences of not getting their A tasks done; they lose jobs, don't get a bonus, lose relationships, and are typically quite unhappy. If you're not really a procrastinator, you don't want to refer to yourself as one in your self-talk! Doing so results in the experience of unjustified guilt, which is not helpful! Instead, refer to yourself as an excellent functional delayer!

## ELIMINATING PERFECTIONISM

**There are lots of self-help strategies**[2] that can help you eliminate perfectionism, but only you can know which methods are right for you. Read through the list of strategies below and place check marks by the ones you think would be most helpful to you. Then, pick out three from your personalized list to work on over the next two weeks. Don't choose more than three. Now is not the time for all-or-nothing thinking! After those two weeks have passed, go back to your list and choose another three strategies to try. Go slowly. Rome was not built in a day!

**1) Compare benefits and costs:** Take a closer look at your perfectionist traits. You may think you're more effective because of them (although this probably isn't true), but at what cost? Perfectionism has many negative consequences, and you may be experiencing several of them right now, such as feeling anxious, guilty, inadequate, angry, or exhausted. Make a list of all the ways perfectionism helps you and how it is hurting you (and those around you), and you'll be more motivated to become a high achiever instead.

**2) Define goals clearly:** Poorly-defined goals are exceptionally difficult to accomplish. Specifically define the goal. For example, it's a lot clearer to say, I want to bring in $500 more a month, than to say, I want to make more money. Be specific in the goal. If you find yourself in a situation where a task needs to be done at work, but the task isn't clearly defined, clarify what is required or expected.

**3) Break goals down into accomplishable steps:** It's best, especially with a complex goal, to break the goal down into smaller, doable steps with reasonable time frames. (We will revisit this principle in the chapter on conquering frustration.) Think about what is required to accomplish the task. Make a list of the sequential actions required to achieve the goal and, then, focus on an action or a step at a time, checking off the steps as you complete each one. As Desmond Tutu wisely said, "There is only one way to eat an elephant, one bite at a time."

**4) Focus on the positive:** Use positive situational focusing – find something positive in everything. When working on a paper, focus on the fact that you're making progress . . . even if it's just getting one page written or one step (of multiple steps) done. The fact that you have some perfectionist tendencies means you can be motivated to be a high achiever!

**5) Avoid the never-finished trap:** Many jobs are never finished – some jobs at work are ongoing, that is, once one aspect of the job is done it creates something else that needs to be done. At home, jobs like house cleaning are never really finished. The never-finished trap is when you set an expectation for yourself that the job *should be finished* instead of viewing the work as an *ongoing task*. For many professional occupations, no matter how hard, or long, you work, there's *always* more to do the next day!

**6) Be patient with yourself/learn from mistakes:** Pick or create a sheltered environment for learning, one where you have permission to make mistakes when trying something new. View mistakes as opportunities to learn. Let's say you have to write a report. First, write a rough draft and, then, put it down for a little while. It's *not* going to be perfect. Come back to the draft, read it out loud to yourself, and, then, make changes to improve it. Often it takes multiple drafts to produce a good enough document – that's normal! During these processes avoid negative self-talk. By shutting down the doubting, discouraged, depressed, and disgusted voices in your head, you leave yourself free to learn and experiment without worrying that you might mess up.

**7) Experiment with new things and fun things:** Try doing something new and different that you might enjoy. Reassure yourself that you might not do it correctly the first time, even if you watch five YouTube videos on how to do it, and that's okay. Allow yourself to *learn* without the threat of punishment! Note any missteps you take and, then, consider how to avoid the misstep in the future.

**8) Reflect on your failures and mistakes:** Failures are learning experiences! A healthy way to view failures or mistakes is to view them as **MLEs** — **M**ajor or **M**inor **L**earning **E**xperiences. Consider what you learned from the failures or mistakes and how that will help you do a better job next time. Many times, the only way to discover how to get something done is by trial and error. In addition, think about the fact that whoever benefits from your work cares more about the result and may never even notice the process.

**9) Increase your thought awareness:** Pay attention to your perfectionist thoughts. At the end of the day, or during some other quiet time, reflect on your self-talk. Jot down the perfectionist expectations you have of yourself (your 'shoulds' or messages about failing). Practice thought-stopping, which you'll read about below. Remind yourself that it's okay to stop being a perfectionist and shift to being a high achiever!

## ELIMINATING TOXIC THOUGHTS

Toxic thoughts are habitual negative statements you say to yourself about the situations you are in or about yourself.[3] The thoughts are toxic because they trigger stress emotions such as dysfunctional anxiety, unjustified guilt, chronic anger, chronic frustration, or situational depression. Each of these emotions are discussed in later chapters.

> CHANGE YOUR THOUGHTS AND YOU CHANGE YOUR WORLD
>
> —NORMAN VINCENT PEALE

Eliminating negative thoughts and replacing them with positive thoughts can not only decrease your stress and also increase your self-esteem. Remember, we feel what we think.[4] There are two types of toxic thoughts: situational toxic thoughts and toxic negative self-talk.

## SITUATIONAL TOXIC THOUGHTS

Situational toxic thoughts are habitual ways of viewing situations. These thoughts automatically make a situation difficult because your focus is negative and often self-defeating.[5,6] Your choice of words and phrases when you speak to yourself, or about yourself to others, can increase your perception of the difficulty of any given task. For example, when you tell yourself something is 'difficult' or 'unfair', it becomes harder to deal with than if you tell yourself it's a 'challenge' or even a 'test'. The two examples below demonstrate toxic thinking about a situation.

EXAMPLE 1:

A client of mine who works in a non-healthcare field took a job that did not have any particular requirements regarding experience. Fifteen years later, he was informed that he had to complete six months of a paid internship like all new hires had to do over the past five years. Although the internship was not directly related to his current responsibilities, the experience would broaden his appreciation of factors that could greatly affect his current responsibilities. He was incensed! He sputtered, "It's just not fair!...It's an injustice...I'm just so angry, I can hardly function!" After thirty or so minutes of discussion, he was able to see that everyone, even those who had worked there for twenty years, were being required to do the same. He also realized he was going to be paid to complete the requirement and that, in reality, the experience might actually be beneficial to him. Then he was able to become positive about the experience.

EXAMPLE 2:

Jane works at a hospital that is now requiring all nurses to obtain a baccalaureate degree in nursing. She holds an associate degree in nursing and has worked for fifteen years as an RN. She was so angry that she thought about quitting her job. She said, "It's just not fair! I'm too busy, I have three kids and a husband. I'll never be able to do this! They've offered several seminars to show how they will help us get this done — I just refuse to go because it's just not right!" After only one counseling session we had together, Jane decided to go to a seminar and learned that there was a local program that offered all courses online to be completed at your own pace. She also learned that the hospital would cover all expenses of course work and even give her one shift a week off (with pay!) to get the degree done in two and a half years! Jane completed the degree saying to me, "I can't believe I wasted almost a year getting started."

Common situational toxic thoughts are described below. As you read through these themes, put check marks next to any type of thinking that characterize your situational thoughts or your self-talk statements.

**1) Negative focusing** is filtering out the positive in a situation and only focusing on the negative or potentially negative. "This is just awful or unfair." When you focus on the negative in situations, you actually become hypersensitive to the slightest criticism or the remotest possibility that something negative might happen. Negative focusing also limits your ability to find solutions to difficult situations.

**2) Polarized thinking** is all or nothing thinking, black or white thinking — there are no grey areas or middle ground. Thinking in the extreme tends to carry over to what you think about yourself and can contribute to perfectionism and intolerance for mistakes — viewing mistakes as failures rather than opportunities to learn.

3) **Overgeneralization** commonly involves the use of words like *never, always, and everybody or nobody*. These are broad, all-encompassing thoughts that leave no room for exceptions in how you view others or events. Therefore, overgeneralization can limit the events or people that you allow yourself to attend or be around. Examples include statements like: "Nobody will ever love me," "I'll never trust an Uber driver again, or "Nothing ever works out for me."

4) **Mind Reading** is assuming that you know what's in the minds of others, that is, believing you know what they are thinking and feeling (including what they are thinking about you). The error here is that the information you have to fill in the blanks comes from you . . . what you are thinking and feeling. Mind reading also results in harmful beliefs that others should be able to read my mind as well.

5) **Catastrophizing** is thinking the worst possible. It is common for worriers to catastrophize. A headache is probably a brain tumor. A fuse that went out running the automatic seat in your car means your car is junk. 'What if' statements in your internal dialogue lead to catastrophizing. Imagining, *what if I lose my job?* when your supervisor says to you that you need to focus on getting in the late accounts receivable from last month. Or asking, *what if my son starts taking drugs?* after you see a news alert on TV about increased use of drugs in high school.

6) **Magnifying** is enlarging the meaning of something. Small mistakes become total failures. Magnifying commonly involves the use of words like *huge, overwhelming, impossible, dreadful, and devastating*. The flip side of magnifying is minimizing. **Minimizing** is failing to see the full meaning of a positive situation or your capabilities, such as your ability to learn to deal with difficult situations.

**7) Comparing yourself to others** is always unwise. When you do this, you make a lot of assumptions. *I should be able to do it all . . . So-and-so can do that without difficulty.* You must assume first that that other person is really doing it all, and you must also assume that she is doing it without any difficulties or challenges. If you are constantly measuring yourself based on what you assume about other people, you're setting yourself up to be disappointed in yourself.

## TOXIC SELF-TALK

Toxic self-talk is another example of a stress-triggering non-essential demand. We carry on hundreds of silent conversations with ourselves every day, and it is the content of these conversations that determines how we feel, emotionally, and oftentimes affects us in a negative way, physically. Isn't it fascinating that it is often easier to think negatively than positively? Toxic self-talk commonly results in dysfunctional anxiety and unjustified guilt. Both of these emotions are emotionally painful and often cause physical symptoms, such as increased heart rate, rapid breathing, shortness of breath, sick stomach, muscle aches, and fatigue.

If you're reading this book, you likely engage in some negative self-talk. Many of the negative messages you tell yourself were likely learned when you were young. We learn toxic self-talk from parents, grandparents, teachers, some churches, caregivers, and even from the media. Your cultural environment when you're growing up can have a significant impact on what you learn to say to yourself.

Repeated often enough, negative messages become habits or automatic. That is, it requires absolutely no effort for these thoughts to pop up. In the classic book entitled, *As a Man Thinketh,* first published in 1902, the point is made that your thoughts are like a garden.

Negative thoughts are like weeds and, unlike beautiful flowers, require absolutely no water or nutrients to grow. [7]

Toxic self-talk reduces confidence and creates low self-esteem.[8,9] Self-talk is your internal dialogue with yourself about yourself. Some examples of common negative self-talk messages that people repeat over and over to themselves include: *I am a jerk, I am a loser, I'm not good enough, I never do anything right, no one will ever like me,* and *I am a klutz.* Most people believe these messages, no matter how untrue or unreal they are. These messages come up automatically in certain circumstances. For example, if you answer a question incorrectly, you might say to yourself, *I'm so stupid.* Your self-esteem is reflected in the silent conversations you have with yourself about yourself.

You may engage in toxic self-talk so frequently that you are hardly aware of it. Pay attention to your toxic self-statements. Carry a small notebook with you for several days and jot down toxic thoughts whenever you notice them. You may notice more toxic thinking when you're not feeling well or dealing with a lot of stress. As you become aware of your toxic thoughts, you may notice more and more of them.

It helps to take a close look at your toxic thoughts to check out whether or not they are true. You may want a close friend or counselor to help you with this. Ask if you should believe this thought about yourself. Often, just evaluating the sense of a toxic self-talk message in a new light helps you in your effort to eliminate it. Also, when you are in a good mood and have a positive attitude about yourself, ask the following questions about each toxic thought you have noticed:

- Is this message really true?
- Would a person say this to another person? If not, why am I saying it to myself?

What do I get out of thinking this thought? If it makes me feel badly about myself, why not stop thinking it?

Remember your toxic self-talk statements are well learned; in fact, they have become automatic. These thoughts can crop up at any time with absolutely no effort. You cannot break a habit by just saying to yourself, *don't do that, stop it*! Thought stopping is a very effective strategy that can be used to eliminate toxic self-talk. The thought stopping strategy is described below. But, before describing the strategy, it is important to emphasize that your thoughts consist of words, and words are *very powerful*! The meaning of a word can be empowering or disempowering.

Take a moment to read the phrases below. Say the disempowering ones first, *allowing yourself to experience the feeling it creates*. Then, say the corresponding empowering phrase and allow yourself to experience the difference.

| COMPARE THE DIFFERENCE IN HOW YOU FEEL WHEN YOU SAY . . . . | |
|---|---|
| DISEMPOWERING (TOXIC) THOUGHTS | EMPOWERING THOUGHTS |
| I can't. | I won't. |
| It's a problem. | It's an opportunity. |
| I should. | I could. |
| I can't handle it. | I'll find a way. |
| It's terrible. | This is the type of situation that builds character. |
| Remember: Allowing yourself to recognize that you have a choice in a situation ENHANCES your sense of control. | |

Let yourself really focus and feel the impact of the words as you say these phrases silently to yourself. Let yourself actually *feel* what you are saying in a somatic (physical) way. It's interesting, but not surprising, that the words 'won't' and 'could' are really powerful. The reason is that, when you introduce **choice** into your self-talk, you are more empowered. Research has demonstrated that **when you increase the perception of choice, you, correspondingly, increase the perception of control** that you have over a situation.[10] This principle is universally applicable regardless of age! When you give a child, or an aging parent under your care, a choice, it enhances their perceived degree of control and makes it easier to accomplish tasks and reach goals.

Even though your toxic thoughts are well-learned, even habits, you can unlearn them and replace them with positive, empowering thoughts. The most effective strategy to get rid of toxic thoughts is using the Thought Stopping Strategy.

## THOUGHT STOPPING STRATEGY

The steps involved in the Thought Stopping Strategy[11] are identified below. Again, your negative thoughts have become habits. It requires effort to get rid of them. Follow the instructions identified below. NOTE: After Step 3, in the instructions is a table presenting examples of common toxic self-talk statements and possible counterstatements to help you get started.

---

When you are thinking a positive thought about yourself, you can't be thinking a negative one! In developing these thoughts, use positive words like happy, peaceful, competent, good, loving, enthusiastic, or warm.

---

1) Identify the negative thought/statement you want to eliminate. **Write it down.**

2) Identify a positive statement you can say to yourself to replace the negative thought. **The positive statement (your counter-statement) needs to meet three criteria:**

   a) It should address the same subject area as the negative statement. (The counterstatement to *I'm ugly* would be something positive about your appearance. It doesn't need to be as broad or all encompassing – it could just focus on one feature you like.)

   b) It should have a positive meaning.

   c) It must ring true for you.

*Always use the present tense, e.g., *I am healthy, I am well, I am happy, I have a good job*, as if the condition already exists. Use *I, me, or your own name*.

3) Write down the counter-statement. Here are a few examples of how you can create your own written list or table of negative and positive counter self-statements:

| Toxic Self-Statements | Positive Thought Counterstatements |
|---|---|
| I am not worth anything. | I am a valuable person. |
| I have never accomplished anything. | I have accomplished many things. |
| I always make mistakes. | I do many things well . . . I learn from mistakes. |
| I am a jerk. | I am a good person . . . I have positive attributes. |
| I don't deserve a good life. | I deserve to be happy and healthy. |
| I am stupid. | I am intelligent or smart. |

4) Repeat the positive counterstatement ten times silently to yourself. Focus on how it feels when you say it. It helps to

reinforce the positive thought if you repeat it over and over to yourself when you are relaxed, like when you are doing a deep-breathing or relaxation exercise or when you are just falling asleep or waking up.

5) Each time you notice yourself saying the negative statement, repeat the counterstatement ten times. **The *only* way a learned negative statement can be eliminated is to learn a positive statement in its place! Practice, practice, practice!**

TIP FOR YOUR
PRACTICE:

*Make signs that say the positive thought. Hang them in places where you will see them often - like on your refrigerator door or on the mirror in your bathroom. Repeat the thought to yourself several times when you see it.*

Changing the negative thoughts you have about yourself to positive ones **takes time and persistence**. The good news is that it's not rocket science. **It's simple!** The payoff is worth it! If you use the techniques above consistently, for four to six weeks, you will notice that you don't think these negative thoughts about yourself as much or at all! If they recur at some other time, you can repeat these activities. Don't give up. *You deserve to think good thoughts about yourself.*

## FUNCTIONING BASED ON IRRATIONAL RULES

Functioning based on irrational rules is a third example of a stress-triggering demand. Irrational rules are rules that have no real benefit to you and serve no constructive or meaningful purpose. Common types of irrational rules are:

*Everyone in the house should hang their coats facing the same direction in the closet.*

*The bed should be made every day . . . even if no one is coming over.*

*Everyone must put the dishes in the dishwasher exactly the same way.*

*The house must be fully cleaned every week.*

Examining how clothes are hung in the closet is an interesting exercise. Put your hands together, interlocking your fingers. Note whether or not your left thumb is over or under your right thumb. Not everyone's thumb position will be the same. If the left thumb overlaps the right, there is an 80% chance that, by nature, you hang your clothes in the closet with the opening of the garment facing to the left and vice versa, if right thumb is over the left thumb. Expecting someone to go against what comes naturally to him/her is expecting them to go against nature.

Like values and beliefs, we typically learn irrational rules from our parents, grandparents, churches, teachers, and community groups. In fact, you probably have some of these people on your "internal dialogue board of directors." You can hear them saying: *Did you make your bed?* or *You must never leave the house without clean underwear.*

One evening, many years ago, I was out to dinner with my mother and a colleague friend. My friend had just been over to my house the week before. I was doing something in the kitchen and needed to get something from my upstairs bedroom. She volunteered to go up and get it for me. When she came back down, she said, "You just gave me the greatest gift ever!" I was really puzzled. She said, "Your bed wasn't made. Oh my gosh, that was awesome. Frankly, I never would have thought you could go without making your bed. There are days I would love to do that!" During dinner, the conversation migrated to all the things people spend their time doing that really don't matter. My friend told my mother about the gift I gave her. My mother looked at me with a shocked look and said, "You mean you didn't make your bed!" I said to her, "Mother, I love you dearly but you're no longer on my board of directors subcommittee on bed making." She just looked at me and smiled.

Remember, you are in charge of your thoughts. You are the CEO and president of your internal dialogue board of directors! We may have learned *many* useful and important things from the people who influenced us growing up, but, if you need to fire or let go of a member of your board, do it!

## ELIMINATING NON-ESSENTIAL EXTERNAL DEMANDS

External demands are oftentimes difficult to manage because we cannot control many things in nature, and we certainly cannot control other people (despite our best efforts).

There are times when you need to say "no" to prevent overload and allow you to focus on what is important for your well-being. Some constructive considerations for "saying no" in an effective way are: communicate in a caring way that you are "not in a position" or "able" to do X at this time, e.g. "I would really like to be able to help you out but I'm not able, at this time, given all of my other demands . . . is there something that I can do next month?" or "I'm not able to take the full responsibility for the committee at this time but I could contribute "____.""

There are, however, four important strategies that can go a long way in managing external demands. These are listed below. Put a check mark by any strategies you would like to implement.

☐ **Set limits.** Everyone has the right to set limits, including you! You may control interruptions during work, or during at-home tasks, by being clear with people about when you need quiet, uninterrupted time to work or rest. You might leave your office door only partially open, limit how often during a day you check your email, turn your cell phone off or put it in silent mode, or leave a noisy environment. You might also focus on one task at a time, prioritize tasks, and be clear with others about what you can take on today, tomorrow, or during the next week or month.

☐ **Say NO effectively.** Saying *no* to a request is often difficult for people, but it is not something to be shy about. It is particularly difficult to say no if your values include being a "helpful person" or you believe that it's necessary to do things for others so that they like you. You might have trouble saying no because you want to show that you are a decent person or you don't want to hurt others. Saying yes when you need to say no indicates that your self-esteem is dependent on what others think of you . . . not a good position to be in! When driven by a belief that you should always be helpful, you will likely experience anticipatory guilt (discussed in Chapter seven) when you think about saying no. The dynamics of guilt are interesting when it comes to saying no. When a person asks you to do something that you do not want to do yet your idealized self says, *I should do it*, the emotion that is triggered is anticipatory guilt. You may not have even said no yet, but you feel guilty thinking about the exchange to come. Guilt is the most motivating emotion for personal change, and, to fix the guilt, you say yes because it is the easiest way to sidestep problems in the moment. It is common to get aggravated later at the person for asking you in the first place.[12]

☐ **Delegate.** Delegating to others is particularly hard for perfectionists and for people who like to maintain tight control over anything and everything. That is, everything has to be done just so, no variations allowed! This all-or-nothing thinking is, in itself, stress-inducing. To delegate a task effectively, be clear about what the task is and if it can be broken down into segments or parts. Maybe you only need to delegate part of a complex project. Do not expect another person to do the task *just as I do . . .* and ask yourself, *what does 'good enough' look like?* Be clear with the person you delegate to about the time frame for completion of the task and whether or not they need to report back to you.

☐ **Manage Expectations.** Being clear with others about expectations is critical. Expectations deeply affect relationships of all kinds. Clear expectations are a central component of any good relationships, whether at work or at home. Lack of clarity in expectations leads to a lot of unnecessary anger and conflict. Communicating expectations clearly can be a challenge because we often assume that people already know what we expect or that others can read our minds (see above on mind reading), even though we know this is highly unlikely. Even worse, there is also a common wish that, if expectations are not openly discussed, they don't exist. **Nothing can be further from the truth.** In fact, if expectations aren't discussed everyone just imagines what the expectations are, and they fill their version into the situation. Disaster! I have had many experiences consulting with hospitals and corporations where there has been a substantial change in the way care is given or in the way business is done. It is common for irritation and anger to be a predominant emotion during these times, primarily due to a lack of communication about expectations. When upper management doesn't fill in the blanks, staff members fill in the blanks in their imaginations and end up getting angry about imagined burdens and insults that may not even exist. These

HAVEN'T YOU SUFFERED ENOUGH?

feelings of anger, and even betrayal, are often a surprise to upper management because none of what the staffers were anticipating was true. All management wanted was for everyone to do their best as difficult situations arose while implementing the change.

---

Many years ago, I did some consulting work for the Indiana Department of Transportation regarding road rage. One issue was the importance of letting drivers know what to expect when there is a major traffic problem ahead. Many years later, most transportation departments now use technology to warn drivers with messages on large computerized signs such as:

**Expect significant delays for the next 10 miles.**

---

One of the best examples of expectation management by a business was this from Jersey's Café in Carmel, Indiana. When you enter the café, before you are seated, you are handed a **WELCOME TO JERSEY'S!** flyer to read before looking at the two menus. Here's what the flyer says:

## WELCOME TO JERSEY'S!

---

### PLEASE READ FIRST

---

**Thank you for choosing Jersey's today; we are glad to welcome newcomers as well as our seasoned patrons. Jersey's is likely different than any other restaurant you have been to in the past. All of our food is prepared fresh from the time you order it. We use no heat lamps, microwaves, or quick fryers in our kitchen. That being**

**said--on occasion our wait times can exceed an hour. We strive hard to minimize our wait times, but with the satisfaction we have received from our current customers and the awareness that the Food Network program Diner, Drive-Ins and Dives has brought us, our business is often times at capacity with a waiting line. Should the possibility of a wait hinder your schedule today we urge you to join us when your schedule permits.**

*Each table has a deck of playing cards so that you can enjoy a card game while you wait!*

I can only imagine the number of arguments and irate customers Jersey's sidestepped thanks to their flyer and their willingness to set expectations.

TIP FOR YOUR PRACTICE: *When communicating an expectation you have of another person, use I statements such as:* I would like for you to . . . *or,* would you please do _____ *before this evening? Communicating an expectation clearly gives you the opportunity to confirm with the other person that the expectation is realistic and for the other person to confirm that they are willing to do whatever it is that you have asked so long as it is doable. It is equally important to validate your understanding of another person's expectations of you. When you hear an expectation stated or implied, confirm what the expectation is, both in substance and time frame.* Let me confirm what I'm hearing. You're requesting that the project be completed in draft form by tomorrow? *Assuming the response is yes, reply with a statement like,* Is by 5:00 p.m. okay?

Now that we have reviewed the various types of non-essential demands that you might experience, as well as strategies to deal with them, let's do a review on paper. It's always easier to learn anything theoretical when you take the time to write your thoughts down. So, let's revisit the worksheet in Chapter two. Reflecting back on everything you've learned in this chapter, you can do a comprehensive self-assessment that will set you up perfectly to internalize the lessons in the next chapters. Use the worksheet you started in Chapter two or start a new one. Take the time to fill in the self-generated demands you experience and, also, identify which values and beliefs you hold that are contributing to those demands. Identify what you can do to eliminate each non-essential demand. Does this require effort? *Yes*, but it's worth it!

| SELF-GENERATED Non-Essential Demands, Values, Beliefs, & Strategies to Eliminate | | | |
|---|---|---|---|
| DEMAND | VALUES (How you desire to be) | BELIEFS (What you think is TRUE) | STRATEGIES |
|  |  |  |  |

## TIPS FOR ELIMINATING NON-ESSENTIAL DEMANDS

1. Eliminate the non-essential internal demands you have identified:
   a. Avoid perfectionism by reminding yourself that *no* human can be perfect and that, often, good enough is good enough.
   b. Avoid situational toxic thinking by identifying something, anything, no matter how small, that is positive about a difficult situation.

   c.  Avoid toxic self-talk by learning and using counterstatements to your negative self-talk statements.

   d.  Avoid functioning based on irrational rules by asking yourself if how you think something must be done is really that critical or if it could be done differently.

2.  Eliminate the non-essential external demands you have identified:

   a.  Set limits on how you open yourself up to interruptions and unrealistic demands from others.

   b.  Say no when you need to.

   c.  Delegate essential demands when you're in overload and recognize that there is more than one way to get the same outcome.

   d.  Delay attention to essential demands that don't have to be done right away.

   e.  Be realistic in your expectations of yourself.

   f.  Communicate your expectations of others clearly.

## SUMMARY

This chapter discussed the most common sources and types of non-essential self-generated and external demands as well as strategies you can use to eliminate them. The next chapter focuses on how to maximize your resources. Considerable time is spent in this book on how to improve your demand and resource balance because, when your demands outweigh your resources, you are setting yourself up for stress. Keeping demands and resources in reasonable balance, or at a level you can adequately deal with, can prevent stress from the get-go.

# CHAPTER 4

# MAXIMIZING RESOURCES

Trust yourself. Create the kind of self that you will be
happy to live with all your life.

— GOLDA MEIR

Congratulations! You're on your way to figuring out how to de-clutter your life by eliminating the unnecessary demands you place on yourself. Chapter three was a guide to help you identify what you have to jettison and what you have to accept as the normal demands of life (sorry, there's no such thing as a demand-free existence). If you feel you need more time to consider what should stay and what should go, take it! Recognizing your self-created, stress-inducing, non-essential demands, which most likely took you years to develop, is no simple task. Hopefully, you've identified and written down your non-essential demands as suggested in Chapter three. Now, you're ready for the second part of eliminating stress: maximizing your resources.

Why bother maximizing your resources if you've identified your non-essential demands and are ready to psychologically let go of them? What's the value of the extra step (because frankly it can be kind of dry)? The answer lies in our description of dealing with stress like balancing scales. If your non-essential demands are on one side and your resources are on the other, lightening the demand side of the load doesn't automatically mean that you'll find balance. It's human nature to ignore, overlook, or minimize the things and people at our disposal that can help us. This leaves that side of the scale too light. Identifying your resources and figuring out how best to use them brings balance and underscores the maxim, no one is an island. You may think you don't have help waiting in the wings, but you don't know until you've looked around with a fresh perspective, which we'll do in this chapter.

So, what are these resources that we need to maximize? We're going to explore internal and external resources, both of which are valuable in equal measure. Your **internal resources** include energy level, positive self-esteem, and effective coping skills. **External resources** include supportive people (friends, family, co-workers, support groups, religious leaders, mentors), money, material possessions, and a pleasant, safe environment in which to live and work.

## MAXIMIZING YOUR INTERNAL RESOURCES

Words and phrases like energy level and positivity are used a lot, but what do they really mean? When we discuss these vital internal resources, are we using meaningful language, or are we using phrases that have lost their intended meaning from overuse? Let's look at how internal resources are described below and see what resonates with you. Put a check mark by any resources you need to work on maximizing.

## MAINTAINING OR ENHANCING A CHARGED ENERGY LEVEL

We all share the universal human need to recharge our batteries. Weirdly, our culture has developed in a way that makes it normal for this basic human need to be ignored. This is a *huge* mistake. Not taking time to reenergize can result in ineffective functioning and in mental and physical exhaustion. Many, if not most, people have difficulty taking time for themselves, partly because there is no societal reward for doing so. In fact, taking time for yourself is sometimes censured and described as laziness, lack of commitment, selfishness, or a waste of time. That mindset is not only absurd but also incredibly unproductive in the long run.

If you view meeting the basic human need to recharge in a negative way and use language such as, *I'd just be wasting time*, when you think about your need to restore your energy, the emotion that is triggered is *anticipatory guilt*. Most people get rid of that feeling of guilt by not doing whatever is triggering that feeling (like taking a nap, reading a book, or taking time for a lunch break). The result is that the basic human need to recharge is not met. Most people will finally give themselves a break when they feel unavoidably worn out or close to exhaustion. At that point, resting or engaging in a refreshing activity is what's needed, but if you believe that you *shouldn't* need it or that it's a waste of time, you will experience guilt while you're trying to recharge.

Rest is not idleness, and to lie sometimes on the grass under trees
On a summer's day, listening to the murmur of the water,
Or watching the clouds float across the sky,
is by no means a waste of time

— J. LUBBOCK

The bottom line is that if you want to recharge effectively, you must experience a positive sense of self. You have to truly understand that your health and general well-being are *important* and that you deserve to treat your body and mind with care. Okay, so here's the kicker about guilt and how it affects your overall wellness: It is impossible to experience a negative sense of self and a positive sense of self at the same time. Recharging your battery requires a positive sense of self; therefore, *if you allow yourself time to recharge and at the same time feel guilty about it* **you truly are wasting time**! Think about that!

While you're considering how to get over your guilt. Don't forget to eat right; good nutrition and health are essential to creating and maintaining energy. A balanced diet, including an appropriate amount of protein, fruits, and vegetables, along with drinking at least sixty-four ounces of non-caffeinated, sugar-free beverages per day, is good for your energy level. There's plenty of information about nutrition online; do some research or consult a nutritionist if you think your diet may be in need of a tune-up.

## ENHANCING POSITIVE SELF-ESTEEM (POSITIVE SELF-TALK)

Self-esteem is a frequently used term that is often not defined well and can feel nebulous and, consequently, useless as a barometer for how you feel about yourself. For the purposes of this book, self-esteem is how you view yourself in terms of your worth and your competence (meaning how competent you feel to perform the tasks necessary for you to live your life well). Your self-esteem is reflected in your self-talk — the silent conversations you have with yourself about yourself. We talk to ourselves all the time. It's normal! Self-talk is all about you and what you think and feel about yourself. If your self-talk is mostly negative, it's an indication that your level of self-esteem is low. Self-esteem is made up of several components, all of which add up to your multi-dimensional view of yourself. These components are:

1) Cognitive - conscious thoughts about yourself (in other words, the content of your self-talk)

2) Affective - feelings and emotions generated by your self-talk

3) Behavioral - assertiveness, resilience, and decisiveness

People with positive self-esteem are characterized by feeling positive about themselves and their ability to affect a situation. It's not about being stuck up or egotistical, it's about liking and appreciating yourself as a person. Positive self-esteem helps you to be:

- Resilient in difficult situations
- Self-motivated
- Able to accept responsibility for your actions
- Open to feeling good about your accomplishments
- Willing to take risks
- Capable of handling criticism
- Loving and lovable
- Able to seek the challenge and stimulation of worthwhile and demanding goals
- In command and control of your life[1,2]

In other words, a positive self-esteem is important for a person to do well and to feel well, Conversely, a close relationship has been documented between low self-esteem and problems like:

- Uncomfortable physical sensations

- Stress emotions
- Drug abuse
- Eating disorders
- School dropouts
- Teenage pregnancy
- Low academic and career achievement[3]

Enhancing your self-esteem isn't easy, and it can't be done overnight. The good news is that there are many techniques you can use to boost how you feel about yourself that have been tested by health professionals for a long time. A few of these are listed below. Try them out to see which ones resonate with you and include them in your daily wellness practice.

☐ **Create and use positive affirmations.** Affirmations are positive statements that you can use to help you feel better about yourself. They describe ways you would like to feel about yourself all of the time. They may not, however, describe how you feel about yourself right now. The following examples of affirmations may help you in creating your own affirmations:

- I feel good about myself.
- I take good care of myself. (I eat right, get plenty of exercise, do things I enjoy, take care of my health, and attend to my physical being.)
- I spend my time with people who I enjoy, and I feel good about myself while with them.
- I am a good person.
- I deserve to be alive.
- I am a likeable person.

Make a list of your own affirmations. Keep this list in a handy place, like in your pocket or purse. You may want to make copies of your list to put in several different places, like your bathroom mirror. Read the affirmations out loud over and over to yourself whenever you can. Share your affirmations with others who care about you. It's okay to share that you're working on being nicer to yourself; if your friends or family truly have your best interest in mind, they'll be on board. Write your affirmations down from time to time because writing has been proven to help in learning new information or behavior. Your new affirmations will gradually become true for you.

☐ **Take time to do things you enjoy.** You may be so busy, or feel so badly about yourself, that you spend little or no time doing things you enjoy. Even if you aren't in the mood, do something that you've enjoyed in the past, or try something new like playing a musical instrument, doing a craft project, hiking, or going fishing. Make a list of things you enjoy doing. Then, do something from that list every day or at least every week. Add anything new to the list that you discover you enjoy doing . . . and continue doing it!

☐ **Do things that make use of your special talents and abilities.** For instance, if you are good with your hands, then make things for yourself or your family and friends. If you like animals, consider getting a pet, walking a neighbor's dog, or playing with friends' pets.

☐ **Spend time with people who you feel good being with.** Spend time with people you enjoy and who are positive. You can and should practice being in control of how you spend your time. Avoid people who treat you badly or who like to spend their time putting others down or being negative about their lives. I know that's easier said than done, but, if you can't avoid those people completely, try to minimize your time with them or find a way to tune them out.

☐ **Take advantage of opportunities to learn something new or improve your skills.** Take a class, go to a seminar, or participate in a discussion group on a topic that you might enjoy. If you're concerned about the cost, many adult education programs are free or very inexpensive. For those that are more expensive, ask about a possible scholarship or fee reduction. Never underestimate the power behind simply asking a question!

☐ **Do something nice for another person.** This might sound hokey, but, before you roll your eyes too hard, give it a try. If this is new to you, you'll likely be happily surprised at the huge effect a small gesture can make. Try smiling at someone who looks down. Say a few kind words to the checkout cashier at your local grocery. Help your spouse with an unpleasant chore. Take a meal to a friend who is sick. Send a card to an acquaintance. Volunteer for a worthy organization. There's a reason for the saying, being nice doesn't cost anything. Give it a shot and see how easy it is and how great the returns can be.

☐ **Hold realistic self-expectations.** What you can accomplish in a situation is not only dependent on your own inherent ability and effort level but also on what a particular situation *enables* you to do. In other words, being realistic means that you also take into account what is humanly possible given the circumstances. Examples of roadblocks to your expectations could be an inescapable noisy environment, feeling sick, or unexpected interruptions. It could be that too many role-related (e.g., as a parent, full-time worker, child of an older adult requiring assistance) tasks are on your plate. Being realistic requires that you be flexible about what is actually possible to achieve in any given situation.

☐ **Cultivate Effective Coping Skills.** The theoretical definition of coping is: "Continuously changing cognitive and behavioral efforts to manage specific external and/or internal demands when demands exceed resources and the situation is experienced as taxing and possibly resulting in a negative consequence."[4,5] In other words, you're coping when you work to manage demand overload by eliminating non-essential demands and when you ask for help, or when you delegate or delay essential demands that are too taxing at the moment. You're also coping when you change your perception of a difficult situation from seeing it as awful to seeing it as a challenge or an adventure.

The way we cope with difficult situations falls into two different categories: problem-focused (direct action) and emotion-focused (palliative).[6,7] Both are important, and both are absolutely doable. Let's explore these two methods, and, as you read about them, think about how you tend to handle difficult situations. Do you lean toward problem-focused or emotion-focused coping?

## PROBLEM-FOCUSED COPING STRATEGIES

Problem-focused actions can be directed outward to change some aspect of what's going on around you or inward to change some aspect of yourself. Efforts to change something going on within you tend to focus on reducing your own ego involvement, reminding yourself of your personal resources or strengths or changing how you view the situation. Common examples of changing how you view a situation:

- I decided that this isn't the worst that could happen.
- I decided there are more important things in life.
- I'm going to focus on something positive in this situation.
- I'm going to view my current circumstances as an adventure and learn from it.

Maintaining a positive frame of mind is very helpful in coping efforts.[8] Problem-focused strategies help define the problematic situation, maintain a realistic and positive perspective, and help to identify the next steps to take. Read the list below and put a check mark by any strategy that you would like to use.

☐ **Gather information.** Gather information about a difficult situation to help define what needs to be confronted and what might be expected in the future. Examples of information-gathering coping strategies are: seeking information from books, journals, magazines, and the internet or seeking information from others who have experienced similar situations.

☐ **Reappraise or change the meaning of a situation.** You might decrease the importance of a situation by saying to yourself, *this too will pass.* You change your thoughts from focusing on *anticipating* a harm or negative consequence to viewing the situation, *in the moment,* as a challenge. I will learn from my efforts to deal with . . . . I'll learn what works and what doesn't. In the long run I will be stronger because of it. Finding something positive in the situation is a very powerful strategy.

☐ **Set limits and/or decrease non-essential demands**. Setting limits and decreasing demands was discussed in Chapter three. You have the right to set limits and to say no. In fact, setting limits is critically important to effectively manage your energy resources and to help you function effectively.

☐ **Express your emotions constructively.** Being able to communicate what you are feeling to others is an important life skill that helps to validate who you are as a person and helps you find solutions to situations that can be changed. Expressing emotions constructively involves owning the emotion with 'I statements' and focusing on what triggered the emotion. For example, I am frustrated with this situation because no matter what I try to do I seem to run into roadblocks. Is there anything that can be done to make accomplishing this more doable?

☐ **Use your social supports.** Of all the resources thought to help people cope with stress, *social support* is perhaps the most commonly studied. Other people can help you think through ways to deal with a difficult situation and offer suggestions from their own experiences. In finding and using social supports, it's important to focus on finding people who have a positive frame of reference and that you know have a history of success in dealing with difficult or challenging situations.

☐ **Use problem solving.** Problem-solving involves clearly defining the problem and, then, seeking to identify what is contributing to or causing the problem. Often identifying the contributing factors takes a while because there are usually multiple factors involved. Once the contributing factors are identified you can focus on what, if anything, can be eliminated or changed. The Work of Worry is a very important problem-solving strategy to use when you are experiencing anxiety and is discussed in Chapter six.

☐ **Conserve energy and allow for relaxation and recharging time.** Conserving energy means making deliberate choices about how you spend your time, including making time to relax or re-charge. Remind yourself that resting is a priority task — not a waste of time!

☐ **Avoid troublesome interactions.** You have a right to choose who you want to be around and what kinds of situations you experience. You can exercise control in any situation by politely declining invitations to events that include people who you don't enjoy being around. You can choose *not* to have lunch with co-workers who constantly berate others or focus on negative aspects of their work environment. This doesn't make you a mean person, it makes you a discerning person!

☐ **Enhance your spiritual self.** Your spiritual self is your life source, your soul, your inner self, your essence. For many, their spiritual self is very much related to their faith in a higher power. Others adhere to a spiritual philosophy without attachment to a religion. Typically, secular spirituality is focused on the individual finding inner peace and experiencing personal growth. Regardless of the type of spirituality any one person practices, it contributes to a sense of purpose, meaning, hope, and the creation, which supports positive relationships. Research has shown a positive association between spirituality and health. [9,10]

☐ **Use prayer.** For a person of faith, prayer is an important problem-focused strategy. Praying, or the connection with a higher power, is a source of strength. Faith-based coping helps you find meaning, feel a sense of control, experience comfort and social solidarity, and find new sources of significance.[11,12]

## EMOTION-FOCUSED COPING STRATEGIES

Emotion-focused coping strategies help diminish the intensity of negative emotions that come with a stressful situation but do not change what's causing your stress. Reducing the intensity of your negative emotions helps enable you to think more clearly and implement problem-focusing strategies that could eliminate the cause of your stress. Emotion-focused coping is used when events are unchangeable or you have not yet learned effective problem-focused strategies. Common emotion focused strategies are discussed below.

☐ **Use relaxation and meditation techniques.** Using relaxation techniques and meditation can be very helpful in reducing the intensity of stress emotions. In fact, most stress-management programs primarily emphasize these two strategies to manage stress. It is during or after the feeling better moments, brought about by relaxation and meditation, that you can best identify and use *problem-focused* strategies to address a difficult situation.

☐ **Use humor.** Humor can make the *un*bearable bearable. When you are able to allow yourself to experience and react to humor — even in the worst situations — you can get some relief from the taxing physical and emotional pressures of difficult situations. Humor is essentially about point-of-view. Great humor sources include stand-up comics on Netflix, old classic comic shows like *I Love Lucy* or the Marx brothers, funny movies, or joke books.

☐ **Delay action.** Delaying action can be a helpful emotion-focused strategy if the delay will give you more time to think through how to effectively deal with a difficult situation. Delaying action, however, is not effective if relied on to avoid a situation that needs attention.

Two commonly used emotion-focused strategies that really are not helpful, and, in fact, can be detrimental to your personal growth and health are:

☐ **Blaming others.** Blaming others for your emotions or difficulties is not a helpful strategy but, unfortunately, is pretty common. When you blame others, you don't take responsibility for what you are feeling or doing, or not doing, to contribute to difficult situations.

☐ **Indulging.** Eating, drinking to excess, and the use of drugs are very unhealthy coping choices. Unfortunately for some people, indulging is used as a comfort measure that can be deadly.

## MAXIMIZING EXTERNAL RESOURCES

In general, you have less control over external resources than you do over internal resources. However, there are several things you can do to enhance your external resources. Review the external resources listed below and see which ones you have at your disposal and which you'd like to work on finding or making more robust.

## SOCIAL SUPPORT

As mentioned earlier, research consistently demonstrates that social support is the great elixir.[13] Have you heard someone say, "I just need some tender loving care [or TLC]," lately? I prepared the first draft of an article on social support in early September 2001 and put it aside, as usual, to read it fresh at a later date. Then, September 11th happened. Ten days later, I was struck, but not surprised, by the amount of social support given to those most closely affected by the tragedy. There was a lot of TLC social support in various forms throughout our country. A continuous stream of information helped us accurately frame the challenges ahead, and expressions of affection abounded. Our safety was, and still is, receiving vigilant attention. There was a concerted effort to help everyone focus on the positive. We were all abruptly, though happily, reminded of what we commonly share – that above all else we are Americans who value freedom and concern for each other. A strong sense of belonging was pervasive. The feeling of belonging extended beyond our country as eighty other countries were directly affected by the tragedy. What an incredible uplift it was to hear "The Star-Spangled Banner" played in London and to see onlookers wipe their tears away! The outpouring of support in the form of caring messages and funding, from countries around the world, was heartwarming. The expressions of support were substantial and tangible.

The unthinkable tragedy of September 11th made daily hassles seem meaningless. Yet, are there any lessons from the unmistakable social support we witnessed that can be applied to our everyday lives? I think so.

The home and workplace are fertile ground for stress emotions. Just as our emotional self-care skills are important, so are our social support skills. Social support is not a cure-all, but it is a great elixir in reducing home and work stress and in increasing satisfaction. We all have needs for recognition, belonging, approval, safety, and affection. Adequate social support that helps us meet demands in difficult situations can help to reduce stress and, therefore, enhance our sense of wellness.[14] Too often in our home and work settings, we, by circumstance or by choice, adopt a going-it-alone attitude. We're often solo acts. But as the quotation above notes, no person is an island.

What does social support at home and work look like? Social support may take several different forms: informational, instrumental, emotional, and affirmational support.

## INFORMATIONAL SUPPORT

Sometimes, what we need most is information. Accurate and relevant information, about a difficult situation, helps us clearly define a problem and turn it into an opportunity, identify how we are going to cope with the situation, or simply establish realistic expectations of others and ourselves. In an information vacuum, imaginations tend to run wild and focus on the worst possible scenario while fueling a sense of helplessness. When those in the know take time to provide us accurate and meaningful information, in a timely fashion, we feel cared about. We can form realistic expectations and identify aspects of a situation that are controllable and those that are not. Discussing expectations and determining what is doable helps to prevent anxiety, irritation, or anger.

It's meaningful to openly acknowledge when a situation is not ideal or is different from the norm – what everyone has grown used to. Sharing accurate information about the status of a less-than-desirable situation makes it possible for those involved to prioritize essential tasks and to focus on getting those done well while avoiding unjustified guilt.

## INSTRUMENTAL SUPPORT

Instrumental support is the provision of tangible goods, money, and services. Once in a while, what we need is dinner out with family or friends or lunch brought in to work. Other times, we need help with tasks at home or work, someone to pick up the house or make that phone call, someone to pitch in with making the family dinner, someone to stand in for us at work while we go take a break.

Mentor or buddy systems are a great form of instrumental support at work. There's someone to show you the way, teach you the ins and outs. Mentors can often help you frame realistic expectations and break large, complex tasks down into manageable pieces. Assigning weekly chores to each member of the family is a great way to obtain instrumental support at home. This also has side benefits of teaching your children responsibility and preparing them for managing on their own when they leave home.

## EMOTIONAL SUPPORT

Emotional support is often provided by others through active listening and acceptance of your expressed feelings. Do your best to find at least one person who can provide that for you.

When members of your family or work group, for example, are angry, or feeling guilty or frustrated, talk about it – use the practical tips offered in Chapters six through ten. It's true that misery loves company, so it's important that you don't get caught up in trying to outdo each other for who is suffering the most. Yet, it is often helpful to have someone who allows you to blow off steam and to help you think through or identify a positive way to look at a difficult situation.

## AFFIRMATIONAL SUPPORT

Affirmational support includes recognition of a job well done and expressions of appreciation. Affirmational support can also include feedback shared in a caring manner to promote learning. At work you might say (or someone may say to you), "You have incredible potential, and I know that you really want to be an expert in XYZ. I found an advanced class in XYZ to be very helpful." At home, communicating affirmations such as, "You did a terrific job of cleaning your room," helps to boost your child's self-esteem. Saying to your spouse, "I really appreciated your help with the children yesterday when I needed to focus on my budget for the new project at work."

It's common for people to feel unappreciated. Applaud the accomplishments of people around you. Contribute to a feeling of togetherness; catch each other doing something right, smile a lot, laugh, and spread joy. At the dinner table, talk about what went right today – even little things no matter how seemingly insignificant. Hold meetings at work to celebrate contributions and successes. The more you acknowledge others, the more likely they will acknowledge you.

## MAINTAINING A PLEASANT AND SAFE ENVIRONMENT

Maintaining a pleasant or safe environment allows you to focus on what's important in your life and decreases distractions. Work on making your home or work environment as pleasant as possible. Decorate your office and homes with pictures and items that just plain feel good to you. This sounds so mundane, but it really does make a difference if you can enjoy your space. Also organize your stuff! Everyone organizes differently, and that's fine. Just know that unorganized clutter often leads to unnecessary frustration.

Obviously, if you're not living in a safe community you have to expend a lot of energy on measures to protect yourself and those important to you. Do what you can to enhance your safety, including moving, installing an alarm system, and participating in your neighborhood watch organization.

## TIPS FOR MAXIMIZING YOUR RESOURCES

1. Allow yourself to recharge. Remember if you give yourself time to re-energize, but think of the time as a waste of time, you're triggering guilt and then truly wasting time!

2. Practice positive self-talk and use positive affirmations to maintain and enhance your self-esteem.

3. Hold realistic expectations of yourself.

4. Take time to do things you enjoy. Take advantage of opportunities to learn something new and do something nice for another person.

5. Use problem-focused coping strategies to balance your demands and resources and/or change the meaning of a difficult situation by focusing on the potential gain and benefit.

6. Use emotion-focused strategies such as relaxation, meditation, and exercise when you need to create a sense of calm or to think through how you can change the reality or the perception of a difficult situation.

7. Maintain a pleasant and safe environment to live and work in that you can enjoy.

8. Use your social supports to help in difficult situations.

## SUMMARY

In this chapter, we explored important resources that can help you manage the demands you experience. Your internal resources, including energy level, your self-esteem, and your coping skills, are under your control. Focus on making the most of them, and it will help you both prevent, and eliminate, your stress. External resources can also go a long way in helping you deal with difficult situations. They include your social support system and establishing a pleasant and safe environment.

The next chapter focuses on managing the second condition that causes stress – the anticipation of harm or loss to yourself or someone or something important to you. We will look at the idea that how you choose to perceive a difficult situation, and the meaning you place on it, determines whether or not you experience stress. The last five chapters focus, respectively, on preventing or eliminating each of the stress emotions: dysfunctional anxiety, unjustified guilt, chronic anger, frustration, and situational depression.

# CHAPTER 5

# HOW YOU PERCEIVE DIFFICULT SITUATIONS: IT'S YOUR CHOICE

There's nothing either good or bad, but thinking makes it so.

— WILLIAM SHAKESPEARE, HAMLET

Shakespeare was right! It's your thoughts that determine whether or not a situation is bad or good. We touched on the importance of how you view a situation as the final determinant in whether or not you experience stress in previous chapters. Hopefully, you now have a good sense of what you can do to get a handle on balancing your demands and resources. Now, it's time to focus on your perception of difficult situations.

Often, you may not feel like you have control of your thoughts because many of them have become habits. It's easy for your thoughts to become automatic – it's like breathing. You're not aware of the fact that you are breathing until you focus on your breathing. Once you focus on your thoughts, that is, what you are saying to yourself, or your internal dialogue, you can take control of your thoughts, just like you can take control of your breathing.

Almost daily, there are opportunities to view difficult situations in a negative manner, that is, to focus on the negative in events or on the anticipated negative consequences of the situation. You're late for a meeting because you had a flat tire. You have to miss a day of work because of a sick child. You're not able to take a parent to an important doctor's appointment because you're sick. Your landlord has raised the rent, putting a strain on your budget. In other words, bad things happen!

As you know from the previous chapters, eliminating non-essential demands, and wisely managing essential demands, can go a long way in preventing or eliminating stress. If you also use all of your available resources, you've got an excellent chance at beating stress. However, there are times when, even with our best efforts, essential demands will exceed available resources. When that happens, it becomes necessary for you to evaluate or appraise what the situation means to *you*. How you choose to perceive difficult situations determines whether or not you experience stress. As odd as it sounds, how and if you experience stress really is a choice! Your initial appraisal or thoughts in a difficult situation may be negative, but they are not set in stone. You can change your thoughts, and consequently your feelings . . . you are in control! *You* decide if you are going to view a difficult situation as neutral, threatening, or a challenge. I am going to shout this essential lesson out one more time. *Difficult situations and stress are not the same thing!* You can be in a very difficult situation and not experience stress! Isn't it interesting how adversity helps to remove non-essential demands and can help you focus on what's really important?

Changing how you view a situation is called reframing. You can change your initial view from a negative perspective to a positive one. Your toxic thoughts, as discussed in Chapter three, increase the potential for you to experience stress. You learned in that chapter that you can replace habitual negative thoughts with positive ones using the Thought-Stopping Strategy.

And now, of course, the inevitable question: How exactly does someone perform the magic trick of reframing? In this chapter, you'll find that the trick (which isn't a trick, merely an internal conversation) hinges on *perception*. We'll learn about three possible perceptions that are most common in difficult situations: *neutral, threatening*, or *challenging*.[1] Only one of these perceptions (*threatening*) triggers stress and the stress emotions. How you choose to view situations, and the words you use in your internal dialogue, determines whether or not you experience stress and negative emotions. Remember, your view of difficult situations is a *choice*. Part of how you choose to experience difficult situations lies in understanding and knowing how to use perceptual inhibitors of stress. These techniques, all of them entirely based on your internal conversation, include positive situational focusing, maintaining a grateful attitude, and the use of humor.

## APPRAISING WHAT A SITUATION MEANS TO YOU

How you view a difficult situation is based on your perception of what the situation means and what it could hold in store for you. This perception is referred to as your *primary appraisal*.[2] Your perception of difficult situations is influenced by your past experiences, your values and beliefs, your current circumstances, and your typical way of viewing difficult situations.[3] A pessimist will be more prone to view difficult situations in a negative way, focusing on the glass being half empty. Pessimists commonly view themselves as being realistic, which makes sense on the surface, but really doesn't hold water. It is vital to recognize that there is the same amount of water in the glass that the optimist views as half full. It's in the eye of the beholder, *or in the habits of perspective* that determine if the glass is seen as half full or half empty.

**Viewing a Difficult Situation as Neutral** - When you appraise a situation as neutral, it means that you're not anticipating a threat or harm or loss, and, as a result, you experience no stress. Your reaction would be, *it's no big deal, I can handle it, I might need to learn something new, but I can manage it.* Typically, *neutral* appraisals are a response to short-lived situations where one or more essential demands can be delayed without harm, and you can identify a resource with little to no effort.

It's common for people to appraise an unexpected demand as neutral when they have the resources to handle it. For example, you're at work chairing a meeting that is humming along, and you get a call that your ten-year-old son is in the nurse's office with a fever and needs to be picked up. You could ask the committee to move to the next agenda item that doesn't require your presence and say that you will return in about fifteen minutes, after you get a family member to pick up your son.

Another time you are likely to have a neutral appraisal is when you have experienced the same, or similar, type of difficult situation before and dealt with it effectively. An example of this would be: David is an entrepreneur whose business is consulting with company executives who are trying to improve their financial bottom line. His work requires a lot of travel, so he is very experienced with, and pre-plans for, delays. He boards a plane in Indianapolis, scheduled to take off at 5:30 am, for Los Angeles, where a critical meeting is scheduled for 3 pm with the CEO of a major software company.

His non-stop flight is scheduled to arrive in L.A. at 8:15 a.m., Pacific Time. A mechanical problem results in all passengers needing to de-plane with an anticipated wait time of at least three hours. David says to himself, *Well, this is just par for the course. Fortunately, I have six and a half hours leeway.* Passengers get back on the plane after almost two hours, the engines are restarted, and then, shut down again for another mechanical problem. After the passengers deplane again, David calls his travel agent and rebooks on a flight through Chicago, which arrives in L.A. at 2:15 p.m. David says to himself, *I need to call the CEO about flight delays and come up with a backup plan if I'm not able to make the 3 p.m. appointment.* David, unlike many other passengers on the initial flight, took the unplanned interruption to travel in stride because he has dealt with delays before. David's appraisal is therefore *neutral*, he does not experience any stress emotions, and happily goes about his business without angst.

While taking risks can be terrifying, the more you allow yourself to take risks the more opportunity you have to deal with difficult situations successfully. Your experience then builds your resilience to similar situations in the future. You feel confident that you can handle difficult situations because you've done it successfully in the past. This increases the likelihood that you will have a *neutral* appraisal.

**Viewing a Difficult Situation as Threatening** - When you appraise a difficult situation as *threatening*, you anticipate that some type of harm, loss, or other negative consequence will occur. The appraisal of threat triggers one or more of the stress emotions: anxiety, anger, guilt, or frustration. The most common initial emotion is anxiety. It also triggers the need for you to activate a coping response to deal with the situation (discussed in Chapter four). There are problem-focused strategies that can change the objective situation or your perception of it, and there are emotion-focused strategies that can decrease the intensity of one or more stress emotions but do nothing to change what's causing the stress. While fundamentally different, both approaches are helpful and can be used in tandem.

Often, the potential for what could happen in any situation has a level of ambiguity. In other words, the situation can turn out well or poorly. It does make sense to accurately determine the potential for a realistic harm or loss. The work of worry really comes into play when you're experiencing anxiety, and we'll discuss this more fully in Chapter six. *For now*, know that, first, you should determine if the anticipated harm or loss is likely to happen. Sometimes, that is really clear up front, but, often, it isn't. When you're facing a situation that clearly has a real potential for harm, it makes sense to do what you can to avoid the harm. For example, choose not to walk down a dark alley by yourself, or take action to protect yourself. When the solution is not immediately clear, it's important to use the problem-focused strategy of first gathering information to clearly define the potential harm or loss, as well as the likelihood of it happening, and identify what can be done to prevent or reduce negative consequences.

As discussed in Chapter four, problem-focused strategies are practical strategies targeted at preventing, decreasing, or eliminating a potential harm or loss. The following is an example of using problem-solving that focuses on balancing demands and resources: Greg is in an overload situation at work with many more tasks and demands than he has time to address in one day. The potential harm in the situation is that his manager will be unhappy if not everything gets done, which could contribute to a lower performance evaluation. Greg doesn't know this for a fact but is assuming, from past experience, that it will make his manager unhappy. The first thing Greg does is to make a list of all of the tasks he must complete and identify the ones he believes are a priority for the day, as well as the tasks that could be delayed without harm. He goes to his manager and says, "Chuck, I'd like to run my priorities for the day by you. It isn't possible to get them all done today." Chuck looks over the list and moves one from the delay side to the priority side and a task from the priority to the delay side. Greg then goes to his office knowing that he now has a manageable day and begins work on the tasks one at a time.

When essential demands exceed the resources you have available (such as time), it's helpful to think of your demand load as a plate that has room for four or five demands. If there is an additional demand that must be attended to, then one of the demands currently on your plate needs to be removed by delegating or delaying. You can choose to view this type of situation as effective demand management rather than be hard on yourself because you're not able to do it all now.

Another example of a problem-focused strategy is to change or reframe an initial perception of threat into a challenge. Instead of focusing on anticipating a potential harm, you identify and focus on a possible gain or benefit. If you don't get the promotion you desired, you can focus on your disappointment, anger or fear. Or, you can choose to focus on identifying where you need to focus to improve your chances next time. Or, you can use the situation as an opportunity to look for a better job with greater promotion potential. You can also focus on the fact that, when you deal with difficult situations and learn from them, it makes you stronger and builds your resilience.

**Viewing a Difficult Situation as a Challenge** - You always have a choice to view a difficult situation through a negative or positive lens. Even in the most difficult situations, like being diagnosed with a life-threatening disease, you can choose to focus on the potential for some kind of gain or benefit. While that sounds incredibly difficult, you don't have to find something *fabulous* about the situation. It's enough to simply challenge yourself to learn from it or let it benefit others. Many who have been diagnosed with life-threatening diseases talk frequently about how the diagnosis was beneficial in terms of helping them have a more positive perspective on life, not to fret over small things, to identify what's really important in life, and to focus on being grateful for the blessings in their life. In fact, it's pretty common for relationships with family, friends, and co-workers to be improved or enhanced.

Sometimes the bad things that happen in our lives put us directly on the path to the best things that will ever happen!

— UNKNOWN

One of the common uncertain and difficult situations experienced by many is waiting for the results from medical tests, like a biopsy, CT scan, or MRI. While you're waiting for results, you have a choice to focus on the possibility of a bad outcome or good outcome. If you choose to focus on the possibility of a bad outcome, you're guaranteeing the experience of anxiety and likely suffering by not being able to sleep, eat, or focus on other important matters in your life. Instead, you can choose to focus on the fact that the vast majority of biopsies are negative, that is, there is no serious pathology present. You can help yourself by doing things that will distract you like going to the movies, playing golf, going bowling, and going out to lunch or dinner with friends. Instead of focusing on next week, when the results are due, focus on enjoying the here and now.

If the result isn't what you hoped for, or even downright bad, remind yourself that there are incredible medical advances in treating cancer and other diseases. In fact, today, cancer is more of a chronic disease than an imminent life-threatening disease. You can practice reframing. Even if you need treatment, such as chemotherapy, there are a lot of potential positives for you. It's a vacation from shaving, you'll save a ton of time not having to do your hair every morning, and wigs today are absolutely fantastic.

A challenge can also be seen as a journey or adventure. I refer to this type of thinking as *adventure thinking*. **Adventure thinking is using language that reflects an exciting journey.** When situations are challenging but uncertain, such as a change in your organization's structure that impacts many roles, loss of jobs, or transfers, try using *adventure thinking*. Every new thing we embark on has an element of adventure, which typically involves some risk. It's like going on an expedition to discover new things no matter how difficult or upsetting the cause of the expedition might be.

A few years ago, a good friend and colleague, who was the chief nurse executive for a multi-hospital system, said to me:

*The change we're planning in how we deliver nursing care is really tough. The new model of care delivery involves quite a few changes in role responsibilities for RNs, LPNs, and Patient Care Technicians. I'm going to be meeting with all of the staff prior to launching the new model, and, when they ask me questions about how all of this is going to work, I'm going to have to say, "I believe it will work well, but I really don't know for sure, we've never done this before." I'm going to feel terrible, and they're going to be experiencing a lot of anxiety and/or anger. Of course, we've done the best we can with the new delivery model, but I really don't know how well it's going to work.*

Many times, when you encounter major changes, you truly have no idea how things will work out until you are on the journey. I suggested that she use adventure thinking, and we discussed how she could frame the situation and use positive language in her internal dialogue and when meeting with the staff about the situation. This is what she said to the staff:

*As all of you are aware, we have been working on a new model for the delivery of our nursing care. As we begin to implement the model, we're all going to be experiencing a lot of changes in role responsibilities and, therefore, how we work. We want to continue to deliver first class nursing care but do it more efficiently. We won't know for sure how everything is going to work until we try it. I know that's a little scary, but this really is an adventure that we're in together. We're going to discover together what works and what doesn't work, and, if we discover that something needs adjustment, we'll fix it and be better for it. First, although we have a lot of hopes about the new model of care we're trying, nobody has a crystal ball with all the answers. Second, this truly is **an adventure that we are in together**. We are going to: listen to each other, ask questions, be open about what is and isn't working, support each other, and share what we are learning.*

My friend called me the evening after the meeting to tell me that she felt so much better viewing the major change as an adventure. Several registered nurses shared with her that they were ready to begin the journey and felt positive about everyone learning together to make it work. Viewing the major change as an adventure was an empowering perspective that was comforting and reassuring to the nurses.

## PERCEPTUAL INHIBITORS OF STRESS

Perceptual inhibitors of stress are thoughts or perspectives that block the experience of stress. Each inhibitor generates a positive sense of self or emotions such as peace, happiness, or joy. The basic principle behind perceptual inhibitors is that **it is not possible to feel a positive sense of self or emotion and a negative sense of self or emotion at the same moment in time**. Therefore, the thoughts or perspectives discussed below are very powerful stress inhibitors. The three perceptual inhibitors are:

1. Positive situational focusing

2. Maintaining a grateful attitude

3. Using humor

Developing skill in using each of these inhibitors will go a long way to preventing stress, even in the most difficult situations where demands exceed your resources (both in short-lived and more long-lasting situations).

**Positive Situational Focusing (PSF)** is a technical term for "the skill of finding something positive in the midst of a difficult situation."[4] Contrary to popular belief, you can be in very difficult situations, use PSF, and not experience a stress emotion. A person who sees a glass half full rather than half empty isn't pretending that things are different than they are – he or she is simply choosing to focus on something that is positive in the situation.

Positive situational focusing is all about concentrating, or centering your attention, on positive aspects of yourself and situations you're in – even very difficult ones. It's about perspective. The opposite of PSF is NSF or *negative situational focusing*. Everyone has the ability to change perspective in a situation. Hearing someone say, "You know, I could choose to see it that way, but I choose to focus on this instead," is an example of having the inherent ability to view the same situation in different ways. Yet, it's common for people to develop a habit of NSF – always seeing the glass half empty. *Developing a **habit** of focusing on the negative in difficult situations makes it difficult to imagine that what you say to yourself, about yourself, or about situations, is actually your choice.* This is a key concept to remember as you move through the rest of this book. **Habits are ingrained choices but are absolutely changeable.**[5]

Thinking negatively is detrimental to your health. It can depress your immune system, raise your blood pressure, and increase your blood sugar.[6] The real challenge for people who have developed a negative perspective habit is seeing that you can choose to think differently. Most of us have experienced people who are members of a work team, where conditions externally are pretty good, who hold on to a negative perspective. It's like Joe, the complainer. He likes to feel like he's a victim. Nothing is ever good enough when someone has a persistent negative situational focus. Individuals like Joe seem to enjoy suffering when others around them are enjoying themselves. Joe probably has low self-esteem and tries to help himself feel better by blaming how he's feeling on others. Oftentimes, a person with NSF works hard to recruit other people into their perspective – misery loves company. You can, and should, resist the impulse to join in someone else's misery-meltdown. Being sympathetic to someone else does not include taking on their negative perspectives. Joining in doesn't make you a good or better person!

PSF is not about putting blinders on and pretending that everything is ok. It's not about ignoring real potentials for harm, such as walking down a dark alley at midnight in a high crime district or eating a lot of sugar if you're a diabetic. It is about realizing that it's your thoughts about a situation that bring meaning and significance to it.[7] The current healthcare system can be viewed from a hopeless perspective or from a positive perspective. A positive perspective might be: If we capitalize on making healthcare challenges real to decision makers, external stakeholders, or persons running for election, we have opportunities to reinvent the way the healthcare system operates in this country. Thinking positively has beneficial effects on your health. It enhances your immune system, contributes to lower blood pressure, and releases endorphins. [8,9]

The idea of PSF is a simple one, but it's not easy for pessimists or those who have developed a habit of negative situational focusing to get. Remember, how a situation is perceived is in the eye of the beholder.

## THE POWER OF PERCEPTION – A STORY

One of the best examples of this appeared in a *60 Minutes* interview Mike Wallace did, in the late 1970s, with two men, identical twins who were dwarfs standing only 34 inches tall. They were abandoned by their biological mother at an early age and, fortunately, were fostered by a very caring couple who taught them to focus on the positive. That is, they helped them learn that although they would face many difficult situations, it was always important to focus on something that was positive. As they were growing up in the Miami area, they became intrigued by the real estate business and, at age 13, set identical goals. They each wanted to be a realtor, they each wanted to be a millionaire, and they each wanted to drive a Cadillac. Wallace was interviewing them 14 years later, at age 27. They both were realtors, both were millionaires, and both had Cadillacs. Wallace talked with them about how difficult it was growing up – how inhumanely adults and peers treated them. They also talked about the difficulties of being successful in the real estate business even when you are of normal stature. Many people just simply wouldn't give them their business because they associated their lack of size with less competence.

It was apparent that both of these gentlemen earned their way to the top with hard work. Wallace asked them, "To what do you attribute your success?" Their response, not in these words, but in meaning was positive situational focusing. They shared several examples with Wallace. In one example, they were leaving their suburban home for an appointment in an office building in downtown Miami. They were in one of their big Cadillacs, with all of its special controls because they couldn't reach the pedals, driving full speed on a four-lane highway, and the right rear tire went flat. They slid out of the car and walked back to the tire – standing there shoulder to shoulder they looked at each other and said, "Thank God three of them stayed up!" Mike asked, "You mean you didn't get angry?" They replied, "What would that have accomplished? We needed every ounce of energy we had to change that tire– and thank God we only had to do that once!"

As these men demonstrated, how you choose to view a situation, what you choose to focus on, will determine how you feel and likely will determine your ability to deal effectively with the situation. Positive situational focusing is not a pretense that life is better than it is – it is instead well-founded. A person who uses PSF realizes that there are both positive and negative things going on in most situations and that the meaning given to a situation is a choice.

The quality of your work life and home life are, in large measure, determined in your mind. You can view your life and your circumstances as a garden with flowers, bushes, and trees. Some gardens flourish because they have been planted in rich soil and are well tended with fertilizer, pruning, and weeding. Other gardens are planted in the midst of a lot of clay and are not well tended. Sometimes, you need to decide that your garden needs to be planted in better soil. That is, you might need to change jobs, change where you live, and/ or change some relationships. When a horse dies it's time to get off – don't complain about it. Just take action!

You can choose positive situational focusing or choose to be trapped in negative situational focusing. It's fascinating to observe people around you and realize that it is much easier to think negative thoughts than it is to think positive ones. It bears repeating Allen's analogy between our thoughts and plants. The essence of the analogy is that if you want to grow a beautiful garden it requires effort: water, fertilizer, tilling, and sunlight. Weeds, however, just like negative thoughts, require no effort at all to grow, spread, and thrive. [10]

## HAVING A GRATEFUL ATTITUDE

It is not possible to experience a negative emotion when you're focused on being grateful for something! Sustaining a grateful attitude blocks the experience of stress emotions because, again, it's not possible to feel a positively-toned emotion and a negatively-toned emotion at the same time. We are not born with an ungrateful attitude. It's learned! We're also not born with a grateful attitude. It, too, is learned. Too often, throughout life, we are schooled in the mistakes we've made, what's not right in the world, how inadequate we are, how much more a neighbor or colleague has than we have, or how much more athletic or fit a friend is. Unlearning that way of thinking can be tricky, at first, but, as with all habits, positive thinking and a grateful attitude can become a habit if you stick with it.

Having a grateful attitude is also good for your health! Being thankful for all you have can boost your happiness, enhance your sense of well-being, enhance your sense of joy in small things, improve your sleep, decrease stress emotions, and improve your mental health. [11]

Gratitude can transform common days into thanksgiving, turn routine jobs into joy, and change ordinary opportunities into blessings.

— WILLIAM ARTHUR WARD

Helen was the caregiver for her husband, who had Alzheimer's disease. It was really difficult for her because he required a lot of assistance. He could no longer travel or get enjoyment out of any recreational activities, and he needed assistance with his self-care, including eating. Although she had help, once a day for about two hours, in bathing and dressing him, it was easy for her to feel over-whelmed and angry about this whole situation. Helen learned to focus on what she could be grateful for, including that she could still hug him, tell him that she loved him, and listen to music with him, which he did seem to enjoy. She focused on little things like enjoying her cup of coffee in the morning and reading the newspaper, enjoying the sunset, and enjoying visits from their family members. Rather than focusing on what she had lost, she focused on what she still had and was grateful for those things. She said, "You know, it really does help to focus on what's positive rather than on what's negative. It does require conscious effort, but it's worth it!"

Learning to have a grateful attitude requires practice. It's helpful to keep a gratitude journal where you document what you are grateful for in your life, both at work and at home. Remind yourself each morning of at least three of things for which you are grateful. It's also helpful to sit around the dinner table with family or friends and share what you're grateful for – in fact, you can even do this in the break room at work. In the car, remind yourself several times of people, things, or events for which you are grateful. Looking around at the world today, there are *lots* of things to be grateful for, including seemingly small things. You can even be grateful that you have toilet paper in the house because many people do not! It's amazing how difficult it is for some people to identify what they are grateful for simply because they haven't really thought about it. No gratitude is too small.

## USING HUMOR

Using humor is also a great way to help prevent or reduce stress.[12] It can be a highly effective emotion-focused coping strategy, as discussed in Chapter four. Humor helps us gain a different perspective on difficult situations. Additionally, when you have a sense of humor works like a magnet. People are drawn to others who have a good sense of humor. Laughter feels good. It stimulates the release of endorphins, reduces the production of the stress hormone cortisol, and can actually enhance your immune system.[13,14] When you feel good, you feel more in control. Having a good sense of humor increases your sense of choice about how you view situations and, therefore, enhances your sense of control. Remember, as you increase your perceived degree of choice in a situation, you enhance your perceived degree of control. You can say to yourself, *I can choose to view this situation negatively, or I can find some source of humor in it.*

There are very effective ways to increase your sense of humor and to stimulate laughter. Here are a few listed below:

1. Post your favorite comic strips or hilarious greeting cards in your office or at home.

2. Watch funny movies, read funny books, and watch comedy videos. (Lucy Ricardo's funny scenes: fighting with a fellow grape-squashier in a vineyard, getting drunk doing a commercial for Vitameatavegamin, or handling candy for packaging on a conveyor belt, are hilarious – just thinking about these as I'm writing makes me laugh inside!).

3. Play games that generate laughter.

4. Spend time with family and friends who can laugh with you.

5. Share funny stories and jokes.

6. Reflect on past experiences that were funny, connect with those experiences, share the experiences with others who can laugh with you.

7. Just smile and start laughing. It's really fun to do this in a group of people as you end up laughing at each other (you can even take laugh breaks at work).

Humor can be learned! The more you practice humor, the more you increase your sense of humor, and the easier it becomes.

## USING THE PHRASE 'CHOICE POINT'

As you have seen in this chapter, you can choose to change your perception of a situation. You carry on hundreds of silent conversations with yourself every day. Right now, you're making comments to yourself about what you think about the content of this chapter.

You *can* change by reframing your initial perception of a threat to instead viewing it as a challenge. You *can* decide to focus on something positive in a very difficult situation. You *can* choose to focus on being grateful, or you can choose to use humor. *You are in control.* It's helpful to think about having choice points.[15] Remember that when you're thinking, you're using words; you're essentially talking to yourself. The content of these conversations not only reflects, but also determines, how you feel, emotionally and often physically.

There is so much in life that we can't control – other people, their behavior and decisions, accidents, many diseases, and natural disasters. We do, however, control our thoughts. The situations we're in, and the people around us, do not control our thoughts. We produce our own internal reality by how we choose to think – the words we choose to say to ourselves.

**When you truly realize that you control your own thinking, you can have a different relationship with your thoughts**, a relationship that allows you not to take your thoughts too seriously because you know you can change them. *You are not your thoughts!* Every situation presents us with a choice of how to view it. Recently, a client, who was learning to remind herself about choice points, told me that she and her husband were waiting in a line of cars at McDonald's for carry-out. It was taking forever, and they needed to get home to meet their children. They began to get irritated, saying, "What kind of incompetent people do they have working here?!" They looked at each other and said, "**Choice Point!**" Suddenly, they said to each other, "So what's an extra 15 minutes – we could take advantage of this time to talk about plans for our summer vacation."

Just like with your thoughts, you have a choice to stay in situations you don't like or to leave them. You may say, I can't leave this job because right now I need the money I make here. Well, that's *your choice*, and it's important to recognize that you are choosing to stay in the job because you need the money. In fact, focusing on the fact that it's your choice actually enhances your sense of personal control! When you choose to stay in difficult situations, focusing on something positive can help energize you and helps you prevent stress emotions.

Another choice point is going to work and realizing that there is more work to be done than could possibly be done in eight hours. You could say, *this is just not ok. I have a right to be upset about this!* You *could* also say to yourself, ***choice point!*** and ask yourself, *what's another way to view this? What's one positive thing in this situation that I can focus on?* Maybe it's that you're in control of your thoughts here, and you're just going to do the best you can do and feel good about what you get done.

## TIPS FOR PREVENTING OR ALLEVIATING STRESS BY MANAGING YOUR THOUGHTS:

1. Remember difficult situations and stress are not the same thing!

2. You can choose to view a difficult situation as a positively-toned *challenge* (e.g., "I will learn from this rather than just focusing on the potential for harm!"

3. When faced with a big change or a lot of unknowns, use *adventure thinking* to frame the situation as a journey where you will learn new skills.

4. Learn to use *positive situational focusing,* identifying something positive in any difficult situation, deliberately practicing PSF so that it becomes a habit.

5. Practice having a grateful attitude daily.

6. Use humor to bring laughter to a difficult situation as appropriate.

7. Practice saying, *choice point*, to remind yourself that you have a choice in what you focus on in difficult situations.

## SUMMARY

In the final analysis, it's your thoughts about how you view difficult situations that determine whether or not you experience stress. You learned in this chapter that focusing on the potential for harm or loss (threat) triggers stress and stress emotions. How you view a situation is really your choice. Choosing to view difficult situations as challenges is energizing and helps to stop the experience of stress.

Additionally, you learned about three perceptual inhibitors of stress: positive situational focusing, maintaining a grateful attitude, and using humor.

Next, we will learn about the specific thoughts that trigger the stress emotions, including anxiety, guilt, anger, and frustration. The next chapter focuses on anxiety. Sometimes, anxiety is functional, and, many times, it is dysfunctional. If anxiety intensifies significantly, it commonly morphs into panic attacks. You will learn the cause of anxiety, the difference between functional and dysfunctional anxiety, and how to alleviate anxiety as well as panic attacks. None of that will be difficult. Don't panic!

# CHAPTER 6

# CONQUERING DYSFUNCTIONAL ANXIETY

What you say to yourself matters!

We're about to get into the real fun of conquering stress: facing and destroying anxiety. Did you just read that sentence and think, *Yeah, right*? Destroy anxiety. Nice idea, but have you *met* my anxiety? If so, you'd be in the majority. Most people believe that anxiety, and its unholy progeny stress, is something we have to muscle through even when we would rather get into bed, stay under the covers, and never emerge again. There is no doubt that your stress experience could be outrageous (or epic, crippling, horrifying, annoying . . . take your pick). There is also no doubt that you can control it because your anxiety is not due to a psychiatric disorder. It doesn't happen

> THE MIND IS ITS OWN PLACE, AND IN ITSELF CAN MAKE A HEAV'N OUT OF HELL, AND A HELL OF HEAV'N.
>
> —JOHN MILTON

overnight, but practicing the right techniques, as an integral part of your well-being, will one-hundred percent get you where you want to go. What are these techniques? Read on!

But first, a recap to prepare you for our next big step: We've covered the **two conditions** that must be present for you to experience stress: **your demands outweigh your resources**, and **you perceive the potential for harm or loss (threat) to you or somebody or something that is important to you**. Also included in the previous chapters were suggestions for how to balance your demands and resources by eliminating non-essential demands and increasing your resources. We also learned that how you perceive difficult situations when demands exceed resources is important — you can control your perceptions. You alone hold the key to changing a perception of *threat* into a perception of *challenge*. You can choose to use stress-inhibiting perceptions such as positive situational focusing, holding a grateful attitude, and using humor.

Once the two conditions for stress exist for you, your internal dialogue (the conversation you have with yourself) determines how you feel, emotionally. Different kinds of thoughts trigger different emotions. In this chapter, we're going to explore anxiety as a main stress emotion, focusing on the anxiety that does not assist you (dysfunctional anxiety) rather than the kind of anxiety that actually helps you (functional anxiety). This chapter defines both functional and dysfunctional anxiety, how they feel, the thoughts that trigger anxiety, the difference between worry and the work of worry, and strategies to eliminate dysfunctional anxiety and panic.

Before we dive in, it's important to repeat this: It is the content of the conversations we have with ourselves that determines how we feel, emotionally and, often, physically. When you are thinking, you are talking to yourself. When you think to yourself, *I'm not smart enough, I can't do it, I'm a failure, nobody likes me*, you damage your self-esteem and increase the chances of experiencing dysfunctional anxiety.

## WHAT IS ANXIETY?

Anxiety is an emotion that can be functional (healthy) or dysfunctional (unhealthy).[1] It is a core stress emotion because its origin is the same thought that triggers stress. Functional anxiety can be healthy when it serves as an early warning signal to pay attention and avoid potentially dangerous or upsetting situations. Functional anxiety tells you, *don't walk down that dark alley*, *prepare for that important presentation at work*, or *investigate nursing homes you are considering for a loved one*. Functional anxiety is a *protective emotion*. Dysfunctional anxiety, however, is a *destructive emotion*. It can create unnecessary suffering and prevent you from realizing your true potential. It is dysfunctional and harmful when your imagination generates potential harms or losses that don't have a reasonable chance of happening or that cause you to spend excessive time worrying, or lead to anxiety, or even panic attacks. Clearly, dysfunctional anxiety has got to go!

## WHAT DOES ANXIETY FEEL LIKE?

Anxiety feels awful, no matter what kind it is. Your body doesn't know the difference between functional or dysfunctional anxiety. The common physical signs of anxiety can include a queasy feeling in your stomach, rapid pulse, pounding heart, muscle tension and tightness, sweating palms, faster breathing, feeling flushed, and clenching your teeth. These physical symptoms of anxiety are a result of the increase in stress hormones that occur with anxiety. When you perceive a threat, a signal is sent to the amygdala, an area in the brain that contributes to emotional processing. The amygdala sends a signal to the hypothalamus, a command center in the brain. The amygdala also communicates with the rest of the body through the autonomic nervous system, which controls involuntary functions, like breathing, heart rate, blood pressure (constriction of the blood vessels), and the constriction of bronchioles (small airways in the lungs).

The hypothalamus is like a gas pedal in a car. When it is triggered by a perception of threat, the gas pedal is pressed and a burst of energy is sent out. The depressed gas pedal is the *flight or fight* response that helps you fight off a threat or flee the situation. In addition, the pituitary and adrenal glands release the stress hormones adrenaline/epinephrine and cortisol. These are the hormones that increase heart rate, blood pressure, and pace of breathing. To make anxiety even more insidious, one of the byproducts is that you have difficulty focusing on anything but what you are feeling and what you are concerned about. You're focused on what you anticipate will happen the next minute, hour, day, week, month, or year, and you are pretty sure that whatever it is, it will be *bad.*

## WHAT CAUSES ANXIETY?

Anxiety is triggered when you anticipate a harm/loss or negative consequence to yourself or somebody or something that is important to you. It is an *anticipatory* thought, meaning that what you're thinking about hasn't happened yet, but you are pretty sure it will. When you are certain that a harm will occur, then the level of anxiety created frequently becomes fear. It is critical to recognize that being able to anticipate something requires an imagination! Imagination is the ability to produce ideas and think about possibilities. Our imaginations can generate both negative possibilities, contributing to anxiety, or positive possibilities. It is not possible to think about something that might happen in the future without being able to imagine. And, guess what? There is a lot of room for error in your imagination!

Uncertain situations can be misread, misperceived, or miscalculated. Any situation that is new to you is embedded with many unknowns. New diagnoses, new responsibilities (such as becoming a parent or becoming a caregiver for a family member), changes at work, or new goals, such as going back to school, can be viewed as threatening or challenging (the good kind of challenging). New endeavors can be perceived and experienced as either scary or energizing, and you have a lot more say in how you feel about new endeavors than you might realize.

Uncertain situations can turn out to be positive, neutral, or negative. You often can't know the outcome. Again, you can choose, in an uncertain situation, to focus on the potential for a positive, or a negative, outcome. When waiting for the results of an important medical test, you have that choice. You can focus on the possibility that the test will be positive for disease and suffer from anxiety in the days you wait, or you can focus on the possibility that the result shows no disease. Choosing to focus on the reasonable chance that the result will be a good one doesn't mean you shouldn't identify what you'll need to do should the result show a disease that needs to be dealt with. But, dwelling on that possibility that things won't work out causes unnecessary suffering.

People who experience generalized anxiety are always focused on the potentially harmful consequences of any situation. That usually plays out as the anxious person plaguing himself or herself with *what if . . .* questions. You know what I mean. *What if she dies? What if I die? What if I lose all my money and have to live on the street? What if I never get into college and disappoint my family?* And on and on. The worst part of this kind of thinking, or maybe the best part, is that none of those anticipations are real yet. Until they happen, they are products of your imagination. When you believe that what you are imagining as a threat is real or likely, you experience anxiety. Your imagination can be a *wonderful* asset if you choose to focus on the potential for positive outcomes, but focusing on negative outcomes is a misuse of your fertile imagination.

Test anxiety is a common form of anxiety for those who take a licensure or certification exam. Test anxiety is caused by focusing on the anticipation of failure or of not getting the score you need. Of course, toxic negative thoughts about your abilities contribute to test anxiety. If you're studying for an exam and say to yourself, *I'm going to fail*, it's easy for other (completely made up) toxic thoughts to creep in. You might slide down that slippery slope into thinking, (as if you're a mind reader), *I always fail* (mountain into a molehill thinking, or magnification), or *I planned to study for eight hours and only studied for four hours, so I will fail* (if a perfect goal isn't reached, then everything is doomed a.k.a - polarizing). All of these thought patterns can creep into every area of life at any age, not just in testing scenarios. Do you have those thoughts about job performance? If you're like most people, you do experience these every so often. To get a handle on test anxiety, you can use the *thought stopping strategy* discussed in Chapter three and the *work of worry guide* on the next pages.

## PREVENTING AND ELIMINATING DYSFUNCTIONAL ANXIETY

To prevent or eliminate anxiety, you **must first focus on the cause of the anxiety**, *not the anxiety or physical symptoms of it*, which can freeze you in your tracks. Since the cause of dysfunctional anxiety is the *anticipation of harm*, that has to be the focal point of your efforts to prevent or eliminate it. The anticipation of harm has two components: first, a **future focus** using your imagination (*I'm going to lose* *all my money* or *I'm going to fail this course*) and, second, the **focus on the potential for harm or loss** (*I will therefore lose my house and live on the street* or *I won't graduate*). To combat this disastrous future-thinking, you need to focus on your *time* orientation or *present* focus and your *anticipatory* toxic thoughts. We're going to explore each of these in more detail next.

**Focus on the present.** Again, since the type of thought that triggers anxiety, anticipating harm, is anchored in the future, focusing on the present goes a long way to both preventing and eliminating dysfunctional anxiety. In other words, stay in the now; you can only control what's happening in the moment. That's why I, and other nurses, often say to patients facing a very difficult situation: "Take it one day at a time [or one hour] at a time. Focus on the here and now." The benefits of present-moment awareness are supported by research⁻ that show that being focused on the present reduces negative emotions, including anxiety.[2] There are a few effective strategies you can use to help you focus on the present, including diaphragmatic breathing, relaxation exercises, thought-stopping, and mindfulness meditation.

**Do diaphragmatic breathing.** Often, when people are anxious, they begin to breathe more rapidly and more shallowly. Because we breathe in oxygen and breathe out carbon dioxide ($CO_2$), rapid, shallow breathing creates a low level of $CO_2$ in your blood. It's actually just the opposite of what you would think; it doesn't create a decreased level of oxygen but rather a decrease in $CO_2$ level. The brain needs a certain level of $CO_2$ to function normally. When the $CO_2$ level decreases, the feeling of anxiety intensifies because you feel light-headed or dizzy and may experience numbness, sweating, dry mouth, and, perhaps, even chest discomfort. The decrease in $CO_2$ level is why people experiencing debilitating anxiety are instructed to breathe into a paper bag – it increases the $CO_2$ level in the brain.

It is amazing how many people do not know how to breathe in a way that promotes relaxation. When you're feeling anxious, focus on your breathing and take slow, deep, **diaphragmatic breaths** – where the tummy moves out and the shoulders do not move up. Diaphragmatic breathing creates a physiological calming sense of self through the parasympathetic nervous system, which puts the brakes on the gas pedal of the sympathetic nervous system and reduces the physical sensations of anxiety. Unlike what happens physiologically with stress hormones, we understand far less about the physiology of the relaxation response induced by diaphragmatic breathing.[7] It is thought that nitrous oxide, which is a short-lived free radical, plays a significant role, but this is yet to be confirmed by research.[8] We do know that the relaxation response slows heart rate, decreases blood pressure, enhances the immune system, and creates a sense of calm. Learn and practice how to breathe consistently using your diaphragm (when your abdomen expands, and your upper chest doesn't rise up with each breath). It's best to practice this type of breathing when you're lying down. Put your hands on your abdomen and feel your hands elevate as you breathe in and lower as you exhale. Changing your everyday breathing pattern requires practice, practice, practice, but it's really worth the effort.

**Do a relaxation exercise**. There are many different types of relaxation exercises: progressive muscle relaxation, autogenic relaxation exercises, meditation, and yoga. I have found the autogenic relaxation exercise to be the most effective. Autogenic means self-created by your thoughts. Since **you feel what you think**, it makes sense that this strategy is very effective. Here is an autogenic relaxation exercise, along with a script that you can say silently to yourself.

Get in a comfortable position sitting or lying down. Make sure you're in a quiet place with no interruptions. Take in three or four slow diaphragmatic breaths. Start saying the following to yourself, slowly. Focus your attention on each statement and allow yourself to feel what you are saying.

*My arms are feeling heavy.*
*My arms are feeling heavy.*
*My arms are feeling relaxed.*
*My arms are feeling warm.*
*My fingers and hands are feeling heavy.*
*My fingers and hands are feeling heavy.*
*My fingers and hands are relaxed.*
*My fingers and hands are feeling warm.*
*My chest is feeling heavy.*
*My chest is feeling heavy.*
*My chest is feeling relaxed.*
*My chest is feeling warm.*
*I'm conscious of my breathing, it's slowing.*
*My thighs are feeling heavy.*
*My thighs are feeling heavy.*
*My thighs are feeling relaxed.*
*My thighs are feeling warm.*
*My legs are feeling heavy.*
*My legs are feeling heavy.*
*My legs are feeling relaxed.*
*My legs are feeling warm.*

The reason you feel warmth (and you will) is that the autogenic relaxation exercise has a parasympathetic response that dilates your blood vessels. Remember, the parasympathetic nervous system works like the brakes on your car. It slows you down. The parasympathetic nervous system releases endorphins, dopamine, and serotonin – all mood enhancing hormones. Unlike the sympathetic nervous system, you have some control over your parasympathetic system and can activate it through diaphragmatic breathing and relaxation exercises. If you suffer from anxiety, try this exercise, it takes about 15 minutes and feels great! Try it even if you don't suffer from anxiety! It will still help you to get in touch with your body and thoughts.

Very early in my private practice, I worked with an MD internist to validate that I could help patients experiencing stress-related physical signs and symptoms. The very first patient I saw was Michelle. Michelle was a thirty-two-year-old working as a CPA in a large accounting firm, specializing in tax law. She came in for a follow-up visit for hypertension. She had been on a low-salt diet and diuretics for two months, but, if her blood pressure did not lower to within normal limits, she was going to be put on an anti-hypertensive medication. This follow-up appointment occurred in the middle of March. Of course, CPAs have high-demand months from January through April. Although she had four years of experience at the firm, this was a very stressful time for her. Starting Sunday evening through Friday, she was on edge and highly tense every day. It only took fifteen minutes to determine that she was frequently experiencing anxiety. I took her through the autogenic relaxation exercise described above, and her blood pressure came down to normal limits. Her MD said that, if she would be willing to work with me, she didn't need to go on an anti-hypertensive medication. The lowered blood pressure was a solid indication that she was suffering from dysfunctional anxiety. Her toxic thoughts included statements like, I'll never get everything done, I'm just so overwhelmed, this happens every year, I just can't handle it, and maybe I should choose a different line of work. Michelle learned diaphragmatic breathing and how to focus on the present while working. I instructed her on the thought stopping strategy, and one of the thoughts she changed was I'll never get everything done. She replaced it with, I'm making progress! She was amazed how radically she was able to reduce her anxiety by focusing on positive thoughts. She also told me, "I'm working so much more efficiently. it's amazing!"

**Use thought-stopping.** When you experience dysfunctional anxiety, you are likely engaging in toxic self-talk. Use the thought-stopping technique presented in Chapter three. Remember toxic or negative self-talk is often habitual and habits can be hard to break! Negative self-talk contributes to feeling distressed or down. The first step in changing toxic thoughts is to become aware of them. For example, common negative self-talk statements that intensify dysfunctional anxiety are, *I won't be able to handle it* or *I'm going to fail.* Consider this scenario: Imagine you are told at work that you are going to have to take on additional responsibilities because of the need to downsize. Your boss says to you:

> *Unfortunately, we have to lay off Jane and Emma, so you will need to assume their workload in addition to your new responsibilities. I understand that this will be a heavy workload, but, with your great organizational skills and work ethic, I am confident in you. We're reasonably certain that, in six months, our bottom line will improve, so we think the increased load will be temporary.*

If your automatic thought in this situation is, *I'm not going to be able to handle this,* then you trigger dysfunctional anxiety. You get home and feel absolutely exhausted, not just from the physical work but also because of all the energy you put into feeling distressed. Instead, you could choose to use positive self-talk and say to yourself, *this is going to be a major challenge – I've handled difficult situations in the past, and I can do it again. I will make a quick determination of priorities with my manager and then determine the best course of action. I will put forth my best effort.* Such self-talk is likely energizing, does not trigger dysfunctional anxiety, and is not debilitating. Worth breaking the negative-talk habit, right?

**Practice mindfulness meditation.** Another strategy to stay in the present and find inner calm is mindfulness meditation. This requires some practice. It helps you focus just on the present and can temporarily reduce or eliminate feeling anxious[3]. In mindfulness meditation, you focus on what's going on around you and your senses (e.g., a pleasant aroma, a breeze, any sounds). You focus on your slow deep breaths. You notice the position of your body. If you notice judgmental thoughts or negative thoughts creeping in, you gently bring yourself back to focusing on your breathing. You pay attention to the present without judgement.

Using meditation can be very helpful to reduce the intensity of what you're feeling so you can think more clearly and deal with a difficult situation more effectively. However, relying on meditation alone to eliminate stress, or any of the stress emotions, without modifying your demand/resource balance, or the perceived threat, will not be effective long-term because meditation alone does not change anything objective about the situation or change how you view a situation.

It is interesting that people who have limited cognitive ability, including the inability to imagine or think into the future, do not experience stress. Examples of people with limited cognitive ability are those who are severely mentally disabled or have experienced brain damage to the frontal lobe of the brain through trauma, stroke, or disease. Imagination is a prerequisite for stress and, certainly, anxiety as a stress emotion. People who frequently experience anxiety have very good imaginations constantly answering *What if . . .* questions. Each *What if . . .* question generates more unnecessary negative consequences.

**Problem-solve to eliminate or decrease the imagined harm.** Again, dysfunctional anxiety, different from functional anxiety, occurs when you anticipate an improbable harm. There are two effective strategies to help you here. First, change your initial appraisal of the situation from an anticipated harm to a challenge or opportunity (discussed in Chapter three). *Hey, let's see what I can learn from this!* The second is to eliminate worry. Worry is a classic pattern of future-thinking that contributes to unnecessary demands and anxiety. Worry is a thinking pattern of ruminating about what negative things you anticipate are going to happen. It is characterized by repeating those *what if* questions such as, *what if I cannot meet my new responsibilities?, what if I fail?* The answers to *what if* questions generate an unlimited number of additional perceived potential harms/negative consequences and, therefore, trigger dysfunctional anxiety. People who worry don't usually address these questions in a calm or systematic way to determine if their worries have a realistic chance of happening and, if they do, what possible solutions could be. Naturally, the more you allow yourself to worry, the more anxiety you're going to feel. The work of worry is a problem-solving approach to manage worries or concerns.[4] Many years ago, I developed the *Work of Worry Guide*, based on the work of Irving Janis[5] to help my clients take positive action to determine if what they were concerned about was really worthy of so much mental energy and what they could constructively do to deal with their concerns.

> **WORRY DOES NOT TAKE AWAY TOMORROW'S TROUBLES; IT TAKES AWAY TODAY'S PEACE**
>
> —UNKNOWN

Why is it so important that you deal proactively with what worries you? Simple. Worry wastes your time, which is, as we already discussed, one of your most precious commodities. Think about this: 85% of what people worry about never happens.[6] Additionally, of the remaining 15% more often than not people find they can comfortably handle the situation or learn an important lesson. Proactively dealing with what you are concerned about can save you a lot of suffering!

# WORK OF WORRY GUIDE

## 1. What am I concerned about?

First it is important to identify what you are concerned about, be clear about it.

## 2. Does what I am concerned about have a reasonable chance of happening?

Much of what we anticipate might happen is not grounded in reality. To determine if your concern has a reasonable chance of happening gather information from reliable sources about the chances that it will happen.

## 3. If my concern has a reasonable chance of happening, is there anything that I or others can do now to prevent it?

Gather information to find out how you and/or others can prevent your concern from happening and set about doing it.

## 4. If it is not preventable, is there anything that I or others can do to lessen its negative impact?

Gather information to find out how you and/or others can lessen the negative impact should what you are concerned about happen and set about doing it.

## 5. If it is not preventable and the negative impact cannot be substantially lessened, then how can I effectively cope with what might happen?

When something you are anticipating has a realistic chance of happening, is not preventable, and you cannot substantially reduce the negative impact, then its time to embark on practice coping. Practice coping involves mentally rehearsing what you will do in the situation should your concern actually happen. It is important to do practice coping in a positive manner – that is, imagine yourself dealing effectively with the difficult situation.

## PANIC ATTACKS

When anxiety continues and intensifies, it can turn into a panic attack. Clients describe the panic attack as very frightening – fearing a heart attack or stroke. Your heart races, you feel palpitations, your breathing is rapid and shallow, you have a terrible feeling in your stomach, and, often, break out into a sweat. The natural response is to try to escape the situation, to flee from it, trying to eliminate the terrible physical sensations. It is the flight choice of the fight or flight response. Your body doesn't know the difference between psychologically running away and physically running away. While, on the surface, it might make sense, trying to run away in your mind, to escape the anxiety, actually makes the anxiety worse by increasing the release of hormones and intensifying the symptoms.

The fight or flight response was first identified by Walter Cannon in 1929.[9] Although Cannon's work was an inadequate description of a very complex physiological set of dynamics that occur when a person experiences fear, his work did form the foundation for understanding fear. Anxiety turns into fear as your perceived level of certainty regarding the potential for harm increases. In other words, you're absolutely sure that what you dread will, in fact, take place. As described earlier, when the stress hormones are triggered you experience an increased heart rate, rapid breathing, dizziness, discomfort in your chest, a stomach that feels turned inside out, and sweating. The body is signaling you to protect yourself from imminent danger by telling you to attack or to run.

Again, your body doesn't know the difference between an imagined threat and an actual threat. Your body responds to what you think! A common way to demonstrate this reality is the lemon test. Imagine that you have brought home a big juicy lemon from the farmers' market. Picture the lemon on the cutting board. You cut the lemon into quarters. Now, you pick up one of the quarters and smell the lemon. Your olfactory system stimulates your taste buds, and your mouth starts to water. (I bet you feel your mouth watering.) Your body is responding to your thoughts, not to the actual lemon!

In the 1980s, I came across the work of Dr. Claire Weekes.[10] She was an Australian physician who, in working with clients, discovered the seminal approach to helping them greatly reduce, or completely eliminate, panic attacks. She discovered that the key to successfully responding to panic attacks was for clients to learn to **accept the anxiety, instead of fighting it**. I found that she was absolutely correct and incorporated her methods into my practice. Here is how to follow Dr. Weekes's methods:

- First, when you experience the onset of anxiety take a few diaphragmatic deep breaths. Your abdomen should expand, and your shoulders should not rise while taking a breath. (If you find this difficult, practice this at night or when you're lying down as it is easier to learn in this position.)
- Second, totally *accept* the anxiety. It's ok. No one has ever died from a panic attack! *It's just anxiety, a panic attack, I can handle it!* **Do not fight it**. Let yourself experience what you are feeling.
- Third, focus on your symptoms – the queasy feeling in your stomach, for example. Try to experience it more intensely while you are still breathing deeply. Surprisingly, and contrary to what you may think, the anxiety will begin to lessen, and the symptoms will dissipate.
- Fourth, when the symptoms are subsiding, imagine yourself floating, as in a pool of water with your arms outstretched or floating in the air.

## ANTICIPATION OF PAIN CAUSING ANXIETY AND PANIC

John came to see me when he was 54 years old. He was the president of a company that he founded in 1975. He was a scratch golfer, a good tennis player, and an avid runner. When he was 51 years old, he was golfing with friends when his golf cart got stuck in the mud. He tried to get it unstuck by repeatedly going forward and reverse but couldn't. While his golfing partner was at the wheel, John tried to lift and push the golf cart from the rear. He felt a terrible pain in his back and had to leave the course immediately to go home. That was the beginning of a three-year stretch of suffering. He was not able to meet his work responsibilities, so his children, who had both graduated from college with business degrees and worked at John's company, essentially took over running the business. The initial medical exams and scans did not identify a structural problem with his back that could be corrected. He spent one-and-a-half years essentially in bed or on the couch in a supine position with pillows under his knees to try to manage the pain he was experiencing. He was, then, referred to a neurosurgeon specialist known for his diagnostic skills. He ordered an MRI at a very different angle from what had been done before and identified that there was actually a fracture in a lower lumbar vertebra on the anterior side, an abnormality that was not healing and could explain the pain.

John had surgery and, after the expected post op period, felt great. Being the all-or-nothing kind of guy he was, John aggressively re-entered his favorite sporting activities. Unfortunately, he was not adequately instructed on how important it was for him to gradually build up his muscle strength before engaging in activities that could strain his muscles. He wound up straining his back only one week after aggressively playing tennis and golf.

When the neurosurgeon had shared the results of the MRI showing the fracture, he mentioned that he saw a congenital abnormality, a bifurcation of the lower vertebra in the sacral area of the spine, which means that John's vertebra looked like it was separated into two pieces. Although John had had the abnormality since birth, it never caused him a problem and could not explain his current pain. But, John began to think silently that the abnormality was causing his pain. He never shared this thought with the neurosurgeon and, during the return visit, the neurosurgeon assured John that structurally everything was fine and that his discomfort was probably due to a muscle strain. John went back to bed to minimize the pain. Although his primary care physician prescribed pain relieving medication and a muscle relaxant, neither seemed to help.

After almost *another year* of being in bed or on the couch, John was referred to a pain management clinic. Over the course of a couple of months, the pain management specialists taught him to regulate how much up-time of activity he had before lying down again. After he came to me, during our first appointment (John's wife drove him to my office while he laid in the back seat of the car), when I asked him how much pain he was experiencing, he said it was at a 5.5 level (on a scale of 1-10). I was struck by how precise he could be . . . not uncommon for people who have experienced chronic pain. Before he had answered me, he looked at his watch. He was very clear about how much pain he should experience depending on how long he had been walking and/or in a sitting position. He had learned well a pattern of *anticipating* pain. John's anticipation of pain triggered anxiety. He tried to fight off the anxiety by tensing his muscles, which only resulted in panic attacks and tensing of his muscles, further contributing to the experience of pain. John's panic attacks were also triggered by thoughts such as, *I will never be able to resume my responsibilities as CEO.* The experience of panic attacks was definitely not consistent with his view of himself as a capable, competent man who dealt with a lot of difficult situations as a successful entrepreneur! It only took seven visits with me for him to learn to modify his thoughts and to eliminate his panic attacks, using the techniques detailed above. He went to physical therapy to gradually rebuild his muscle strength and, after two months, was able to resume his responsibilities as CEO of his company. This is the power of the techniques and tools in this book!

## TIPS TO ELIMINATE DYSFUNCTIONAL ANXIETY AND PANIC ATTACKS

1. Accept the anxiety. Own it. It's ok. Focus on your symptoms. (Do *not* run from your symptoms!)

2. Focus on the present.

3. Use diaphragmatic breathing.

4. Use a relaxation strategy of your choice.

5. Use the thought stopping technique.

6. Use the Work of Worry Guide.

## SUMMARY

1. Dysfunctional anxiety can be a very disabling stress emotion that dramatically reduces your ability to function. It is caused by *anticipating* some kind of harm or loss.

2. There are two types of anxiety: functional (healthy) and dysfunctional (unhealthy). This chapter covered anxiety, including what it feels like, with an emphasis on dysfunctional

anxiety. Dysfunctional anxiety can intensify into panic attacks that are even more disabling.

3.  To prevent or eliminate dysfunctional anxiety:
    *   Focus on the present
    *   Use diaphragmatic breathing
    *   Use a relaxation exercise
    *   Use the thought-stopping technique
    *   Use the Work of Worry Guide

4.  To eliminate a panic attack:
    *   Do diaphragmatic breathing
    *   Focus on the present
    *   Focus on your symptoms — do *not* try to run away from your anxiety symptoms. Accept the symptoms
    *   Use positive self-talk: *I've got this. I can deal with this. These feelings will pass.*

The next chapter focuses on the stress emotion of unjustified guilt. Just like dysfunctional anxiety, unjustified guilt can be very debilitating.

# CHAPTER 7

# CONQUERING UNJUSTIFIED GUILT

I don't recall buying a ticket for my guilt trip.

Guilt is a common emotion that serves a meaningful personal growth purpose, when it is justified. Guilt is justified when you need to learn from some act of wrongdoing you committed. Guilt is unjustified when you blame yourself for something that you did not cause or when you hold yourself up to unrealistic expectations. This unjustified guilt is devastating and harmful. This chapter explores what kind of thoughts trigger unjustified guilt and what distinguishes it from justified guilt. We will focus on unjustified guilt as it is the more harmful (and common) form of guilt, and we will explore strategies to prevent and alleviate unjustified guilt. As we will discuss, to alleviate unjustified guilt it is important to accurately understand the cause of it.

## WHAT IS GUILT?

Guilt is a stress emotion that never feels good and can be quite painful. The source of guilt for each of us is found in our values, as we discussed in Chapters two and three. Your values determine how you desire to be in your social and work roles as a parent, spouse, daughter/son, friend, nurse, doctor, administrator, attorney, CEO, engineer, financial advisor, etc. Your values dictate how you act and react, and, when you violate your values, the emotion of guilt is triggered.[1]

## WHAT DOES GUILT FEEL LIKE?

Guilt is frequently a painful emotion and is commonly accompanied by physical symptoms, such as a heavy chest, a sick or queasy stomach, or a feeling of butterflies in your stomach. In my practice, I've seen clients who have had very significant gastrointestinal problems, such as diarrhea, constipation, abdominal pain, and indigestion, as a result of feeling chronic guilt.

## OUR VALUES - A CAUSE OF GUILT

Guilt is triggered by thinking that you have done something that goes against your values (your standards for how you think you should think, feel, and behave). As explained in Chapter two, values are imperatives for action — we are driven to think, feel, and behave consistent with our values. Values, by definition, are inherently idealistic. That is, values represent the very best of how we want to be, our standards. Values are principally learned from social interactions with family, significant others, places of worship, and school. Our values help keep us on the straight and narrow; they are barometers for our behavior. The fact that values are inherently idealistic is positive because we are driven to continually improve. On the other hand, we can have the *false belief* that how we desire to be is inherently realistic and therefore is always achievable regardless of circumstances.[2]

There are different types of values. Some values represent an enduring quality, such as honesty and kindness. These values are typically shared within a society or community. Other values are instrumental[3], or functional, in nature and are more specific in shaping how a person desires to be in various roles (e.g., mother, father, engineer, lawyer, nurse, teacher, salesperson, etc.). Your answers to the questions like, *what does it look like to be a good mother or father?* represent your functional values. Again, values are imperatives for action — values drive you to think, feel, and behave in certain ways. When you do something that does not measure up to your values, or how you desire to be (often said in 'should' statements), the resulting emotion is guilt.

## TYPES OF GUILT

There are two types of guilt, justified and unjustified. Justified guilt supports personal growth and promotes behavior that is consistent with cultural and social norms and laws. Your values serve an important role as your conscience. Unjustified guilt, on the other hand, is a stress emotion that is debilitating. It stifles personal growth by getting you stuck in a pattern of negative self-talk, self-punishment, and low self-esteem.

**YOUR VALUES REPRESENT YOUR IDEAL SELF!**

| TWO TYPES OF GUILT | |
|---|---|
| **JUSTIFIED** | **UNJUSTIFIED** |
| Some type of harm/loss occurred | Blaming yourself for something you |
| You caused the harm/loss | couldn't foresee or didn't cause: |
| Harm was foreseeable and preventable | Decisional regret |
| | Controllability fallacy |
| | Misattribution of cause |
| | Idealistic expectations |

## JUSTIFIED GUILT

Justified guilt occurs when a harm or loss has occurred that was foreseeable and preventable by you. When justified, guilt can indeed promote personal growth. You eliminate justified guilt by taking responsibility for what happened, accepting the past as unchangeable, and learning from the experience to improve your behavior next time. In fact, learning is the *desired* outcome of justified guilt. Our society, and many others, expects a person to experience guilt when harm is caused that was foreseeable and preventable. The individual can, then, learn from and change future behavior as a result of the experience.

> FORGIVING YOURSELF IS AS IMPORTANT AS FORGIVING OTHER PEOPLE. GUILT IS TOXIC IF YOU RUMINATE ON IT OVER AND OVER.

There is little sympathy for a criminal who experiences no guilt or remorse for his or her actions because that person is openly rejecting the values of the society and is likely to continue to do so.

Guilt can also be experienced in an anticipatory sense, not just in the aftermath of wrongdoing. All you have to do is just *think* about doing something that goes against your values, and you experience a twinge of guilt. Anticipatory guilt really helps us to stay in line. Guilt, in this sense, can be thought of as your *conscience*. *Anticipatory guilt is the most common reason people say yes to a request to do something that they either do not want to do or really do not have time to do.* Guilt is the most motivating emotion

> **ANTICIPATORY GUILT: YOU SAY "YES" WHEN YOU NEED TO SAY "NO."**

for change. When you anticipate saying no (because it is really best for you), but saying yes is more consistent with your values, anticipatory guilt often leads you to say *yes*. Often, after you say yes, when the most beneficial response would have been no, you feel irritation or anger at yourself or at the other person for asking you in the first place (when they should have known that you are overloaded).

Some examples of social situations that trigger justified guilt include forgetting an important birthday, saying something to a friend that hurts him or her, not keeping in touch with an elderly parent, and putting yourself in a precarious situation that results in a negative outcome that was avoidable (like going to a party with underage drinking or where illegal drugs will be used). Violating your own ethical or moral code also results in justified guilt. If you have violated your personal standards (e.g., told a significant lie, cheated on an exam, drunk too much alcohol, or cheated on your spouse), you experience justified guilt. When you are caught doing something wrong that violates your values/standards, the emotion that you experience is shame. Shame is a painful feeling of humiliation. Shame can fundamentally affect a person's sense of self-worth and contribute to drug addiction and suicidal thoughts.[4]

The absolute best way to deal with justified guilt is to accept the responsibility for what happened and ask yourself, *What can I learn from this situation and what can I do to prevent it from happening again?* Be specific about what you can learn and how to prevent it from happening again. If you drank too much alcohol at a party, and that contributed to you causing harm, it's fairly clear what you need to learn: Consuming too much alcohol can lead to negative outcomes. To prevent it from happening again, you decide to drink in moderation, not to drink at all, or avoid parties where you are tempted to drink too much. Once you truly learn from a justified guilt situation, forgiving yourself is a critically important aspect of healing.

## UNJUSTIFIED GUILT

Unjustified guilt is triggered by four circumstances: **decisional regret, controllability fallacy, misattributed cause,** and **idealistic expectations**. Each of these circumstances generates unrealistic thoughts: *I should have . . . ., I should be . . . .*

**Decisional regret** is when a person blames him or herself for a decision that led to a negative outcome that could *not* be foreseen. Decisional regret leads to feelings of unjustified guilt. It might be great if we could know the outcome of every decision we make before we make it, but that is just not possible. An example of decisional unjustified guilt is if a person leaves a good job for what seems like a much better and more lucrative job, only to find out that he or she was not told about the significant financial problems the new company was about to encounter, which could lead to staff layoffs. We all make the best decisions we can, given the information and the capabilities we have at the time. When you experience unjustified guilt based on a decision you made, it's not healthy to punish yourself based on hindsight, also known as *rear view mirror thinking*. Guilt is not justified if the outcome wasn't foreseeable or preventable. Don't beat yourself up! Just learn from it!

The **Controllability Fallacy** is believing you can control something or someone you can't. Particularly difficult beliefs are the following:

*I should be able to control that other person.*

*I should have been able to change the situation or prevent that from happening*

*I should be able to make that person happy.*

*I should be able to make the external pressures on the company go away.*

**IT'S HUMANLY IMPOSSIBLE TO CONTROL OTHER PEOPLE'S FEELINGS . . . YOU ARE NOT RESPONSIBLE FOR SOMEONE ELSE'S HAPPINESS!**

These types of 'should' statements are grounded in a belief that you should be able to control what is *not* controllable.

Thinking that you should be able to control the uncontrollable can cause chronic unjustified guilt and contributes to poor self-esteem and situational depression (covered in Chapter ten). First of all, *you* are *not responsible* for someone else's feelings, including their happiness! Secondly, in business or task-related situations, all you can do is the best you can do. It is humanly impossible to control external variables. Let me repeat that. *It is impossible to control external variables.* We all know this to be true, but guilt can override our understanding of that very basic fact! The best you can do is to make contingency plans for known possibilities, for example, the possibility that something might interrupt or change your income, increase your expenses, or stop you from completing a critical task within a specified time frame.

**Misattribution of Cause** is incorrectly assigning a particular cause to an undesirable outcome. An important determinant of whether or not you experience unjustified guilt is the attribution you make for a situation, that is, the reason for or cause of a situation. Believing that you caused something that, in reality, you did not cause, yet feel responsible for, results in unjustified guilt. An example would be a mother who incorrectly blames herself for her child's grave illness because she didn't eat a healthy enough diet during pregnancy. Recognizing that the assignment of cause is incorrect, or not grounded in reality, is an essential step in eliminating unjustified guilt which results from a misattribution of cause.

> ATTRIBUTING YOUR SUCCESS TO LUCK MAKES YOU VULNERABLE TO ANXIETY THE NEXT TIME YOU WANT TO SUCCEED!

Early research in the development of attribution theory was conducted by Bernard Weiner and was focused on the attributions of achievement, success and failure. [5] In the early 1970s, women and men tended to be significantly different in their attributions for success and failure. Most women attributed success to luck. *I was born to the right family. I happened to go to the right school. I happened to marry the right man. By chance, I was at the right place at the right time.* **Such an attribution would make you vulnerable to anxiety the next time you wanted to succeed because nothing about the**

**situation would be controllable**. Men, on the other hand, more often attributed success to ability. *I succeeded because of my inherent ability.* An attribution to ability makes you less vulnerable to anxiety and guilt in uncertain situations if you are confident in your ability.

In the 1970s women tended to attribute failure to the lack of ability. This attribution makes you vulnerable to feeling as though you are not worthy, and furthermore makes you vulnerable to unjustified guilt. Men, on the other hand, typically attributed failure to task difficulty. *No man could have accomplished that!* Men most commonly make the same attribution for failure today.

Over the last decades, the attribution for success by women has changed, indicating that attributions for success and failure are learned! Women now more commonly attribute success to effort. This attribution is quite positive and helps to generate a feeling of controllability in future efforts to succeed. The very best attribution is a combination of ability and effort. Men still tend to attribute success to ability.

|  | INTERNAL | EXTERNAL |
|---|---|---|
| **STABLE** | ABILITY | TASK DIFFICULTY |
| **UNSTABLE** | EFFORT | LUCK |

Of course, it's important to appropriately attribute failure to lack of effort when that is the case so that you can learn from it and put forth sufficient effort the next time you want to succeed. But, it is unfortunate that today most women still inaccurately attribute failure to lack of ability. Thus, there is the continued vulnerability for the experience of unjustified guilt. The most accurate attribution for non-ideal situations where it is impossible to get it all done is *task difficulty.*

**Idealistic Expectations** are perhaps the most common cause of unjustified guilt. When a person holds unrealistic self-expectations, such as, *I should be able to do it all despite the circumstances,* unjustified guilt results. It's critical to recognize and accept that **no one can be *all* that they desire to be in a situation that does not enable it.** Believing that your values are inherently realistic generates the personal expectation that *I should be able to do it all despite the circumstances.* Yet, **no human being can be ideal in situations that are not ideal**. The following two examples illustrate this concept.

Mary Ann is a 34-year-old single mother of two children, ages eight and eleven. She works full-time as a staff nurse. Her husband was killed in a car crash three years ago and had a life insurance policy that helped soften the financial blow of not having two incomes, but Mary Ann still needed to work. She tried every day to be her ideal as a mother, home care taker and nurse – she thinks that she should be able to do it all and do it well. She constantly feels overwhelmed and guilty because she thinks that she isn't good at anything. She rated her stress level as very high and came to see me because *"I'm just miserable!,"* To eliminate her stress, she had to first address her unjustified guilt so that she could then go into demand/ resource management mode.

We first worked on her false belief that she "should be able to do it all" despite the circumstances. You'll get a good sense of what she expected of herself when we address her demand load. She was engaging in a lot of negative self-talk: "I'm not good at anything"; "I'm not being the mother I want to be"; "I love my work as a nurse but I'm only existing at work – I'm just too tired". Her unjustified guilt was wearing her down. After discussing the realities of what was humanly possible for one person to do in her situation Mary

Ann was able to recognize that what she was expecting of herself was totally unrealistic. She was then ready to closely examine her demands and resources.

To address feeling overwhelmed, she changed her language from, *I'm feeling overwhelmed,* to *I'm feeling overloaded.* Mary Ann identified the non-essential demands she was placing on herself, eliminated them and learned to use her resources more effectively. Specifically, in terms of non-essential demands, she:

- Eliminated the perceived need to clean her house thoroughly every week and enlisted her children in helping with chores to keep the house reasonably straight,
- Eliminated her perceived need to fix her children three balanced meals a day and enlisted their help in making their own school lunches the night before and helping with dinner and dishes in the evening,
- Eliminated daily thoughts about what to make for dinner by using one of her days off to plan meals for the week and had the children put meals in a freezer bag to be put in the crockpot for dinner,
- Eliminated her toxic thoughts about being an inadequate mother (*I'm failing as a mother. I just can't do it all. I can't handle it.*) by using the thought-stopping strategy, and
- Eliminated her perceived need to say yes to requests to do extra shifts at work or to helping with activities at church. She learned to set limits on external demands by communicating clearly about what was manageable for her. "Given my current demand load, I'm able to help by making a cake for the event but doing more would be very difficult."

Mary Ann learned to make better use of her resources. She:

- Enlisted her in-laws in taking her children one evening a week so she could treat herself to an evening out with friends to recharge her batteries,
- Enlisted parents of her children's friends to carpool for sports activities,
- Enlisted her brother to be more engaged with her son and his sports activities, and
- Used positive self-statements such as, *it really is amazing how well I'm dealing with a difficult situation* and *my children are learning how to be responsible in contributing to our family and taking care of themselves.*

Mary Ann was able to eliminate non-essential demands and to use her resources more effectively. She was able to recognize that she was actually doing a great job in a much less than ideal situation which greatly contributed to her sense of well-being. Eliminating her unjustified guilt and using positive self-talk made all the difference contributing to a sense of joy in her everyday life. "It's absolutely unbelievable how much better I feel and how much more enjoyment I'm getting out of my children and just everyday life."

A personal example is while working as a faculty member teaching in the master's degree program in the 1970s there was a critical shortage of registered nurses. Today, there is a lot of talk about an anticipated shortage of nurses; however, the situation today is in no way as dire as it was in the early-seventies. The Vice President of Nursing at a local large tertiary hospital came over to the Indiana University School of Nursing and asked if there were any faculty and graduate students who could work as staff nurses. I chose to do some shift work. I hadn't done any bedside nursing for over seven years and my teaching in the graduate program did not focus on in-patient care. Almost everything had changed in terms of medications and medical treatments. My ideal as a nurse encompasses a lot more than administering medications and medical treatments safely and therapeutically — it also includes meeting all of the nursing care needs of patients, including their psychosocial needs. I used to joke that to enable me to be all that I desire to be as a nurse, the ideal situation would be

**EXPECTING TO ACCOMPLISH WHAT IS HUMANLY IMPOSSIBLE DOESN'T CHANGE THE IMPOSSIBLE TO POSSIBLE – IT ONLY CAUSES UNNECESSARY STRESS.**

me and three patients – two of whom were capable of doing most of their own physical care.

Needless to say, that wasn't the situation. All I really had time to do during my eight-hour shift was the administering of medications and medical treatments to eight patients who were very sick. Because I was not confident in my knowledge of all of the medications and treatments, I spent a lot of time checking and double-checking and seeking instruction from experienced RNs on how to do a few of the medical treatments that were new to me. I would take me 1 hour at the end of a shift just to finish my charting. After each shift, I left, saying silently to myself, *Brenda, you are absolutely incredible! You were here for eight hours and didn't harm anybody!* This thought made me smile — a critical principle to all who are nurses is "do no harm." Other nurses commonly left their shifts feeling terrible because of all they couldn't get done in a situation where it was humanly impossible to do it all. I was aware of all that I would have liked to have done but could not do — but I knew that I needed to focus on what was done, not what was left undone. Over time, as I completed more shifts, I was able to do more — but I was never able to meet my ideal.

I have helped many individuals identify their bare minimum expectations of achievement for days that are incredibly hectic with many interruptions. I refer to this type of a day as a *MASH Day* (named after the *M\*A\*S\*H* television show about a makeshift emergency room under the worst possible conditions during the Korean War). A *Mash Day* is the opposite of an ideal day. It is a difficult day when Mom or Dad is stretched to the limit, and the focus is simply getting the bare essentials done. **When everyone knows the Mash Day expectations, those expectations can easily be communicated in the moment.** On *Mash Days,* it's important to focus on how incredible it is that you were able to accomplish what you did![6]

Expecting yourself to be ideal in situations that are not ideal not only triggers unjustified guilt, it is also a primary cause of burnout. Since values are imperatives for action, you are driven to try to figure it out, work harder, or get less sleep because you feel you should be able to do it!

## TIPS FOR PREVENTING UNJUSTIFIED GUILT

The experience of unjustified guilt is a good example of self-generated non-essential demands emanating from false beliefs and your idealistic values that make you vulnerable to an unnecessary and debilitating stress emotion. How you desire to be, driven by your values and beliefs, represents your ideal self and generates *I should* statements that trigger guilt: I *should have done . . ., I shouldn't have done . . ., I should be able to . . .* The corrective self-care strategies to avoid unjustified guilt are:

1. Recognize that the situation you are in is not ideal.

2. Set priorities (the parts of your ideal that are the most important and doable given the circumstances).

3. Celebrate at the end of the day that you did the best you could do, while focusing on what you were able to get done.

It is a strange phenomenon that most of us, while in difficult situations, focus on what we *didn't* get done rather than on how remarkable it is that we were able to accomplish what we did. Leaving work after a horrendous day, saying to yourself, *I didn't do a good job today; there's so much I didn't get done,* triggers unjustified guilt. An alternative self-talk statement is, *I worked hard for eight hours; I got a lot accomplished and the most important things were done.* Focusing on what you didn't get done and engaging in negative self-talk, when there is too much to do, accomplishes nothing productive. Expecting to accomplish what is humanly impossible doesn't change the impossible to possible – it only causes unnecessary stress.

## TIPS FOR ELIMINATING UNJUSTIFIED GUILT

1. Recognize that you make the best decisions possible given the information you have and the circumstances you're in.

2. Accept the fact that it is not possible to control other people and their happiness.

3. Make correct attributions for when you're not able to measure up to your ideal, such as lack of effort or task difficulty.

4. Recognize that your values represent your ideal, and the ideal is only achievable in ideal situations.

## SUMMARY

Guilt can be a very beneficial emotion in terms of keeping us in line, serving as our conscience, and learning from situations in which you have caused a harm or loss. Guilt is commonly a motivating emotion for behavior change and, as such, is quite powerful. But when guilt is unjustified, it is a stress emotion that can be very harmful to your self-esteem and how you feel physically. It is important that you are kind to yourself and do not have unreasonable expectations for what you can do and who you can be. Be the best you can be given the circumstances of your situation. Don't try to control the uncontrollable in your external environment or in other people . . . if you do, you're doomed for misery.

The next chapter focuses on anger. Like guilt, there are two types of anger: situational anger (that can be very beneficial) and chronic anger (that is a debilitating stress emotion).

# CHAPTER 8

# CONQUERING CHRONIC ANGER

Anger is an acid that can do more harm to the vessel in which it is stored
than to anything on which it is poured.

— MARK TWAIN

As most of us know quite well, there's angry and then there's ANGRY! We experience anger on a continuum that starts with some form of irritation and can escalate to full-blown rage. One of the challenges we all face is managing our anger when we encounter situations that can take us from calm and collected to red-faced yelling. While it can feel good to vent when you've "had it up to *here*," the reality is that getting angry with any regularity is, in practice, a bad idea. Not only does it negatively impact your relationships with other people, but also when you allow yourself to get caught up in frequent anger, *you're giving up your opportunity to experience joy and negatively impacting your health.* Anger is most often experienced in interpersonal situations but can also be experienced in situations that are impersonal, such as watching the TV news or attempting to work with a piece of equipment that is malfunctioning.

## WHAT IS ANGER?

Anger is an emotion and, like the other emotions discussed in this book, is normal. There are two types of anger, situational and chronic. Situational anger can be healthy if it's experienced for a short period of time and is expressed and dealt with appropriately. When anger is chronic it is a *stress* emotion and can be physically debilitating and can even destroy personal relationships. Anger is commonly experienced as an emotion brought about by another person's actions or what they say ("How could you say that I've never done anything for you. That's garbage!"). It can also be in an institutional context, such as being angry with a company or organization ("I can't stand the outrageous way that company treats its employees!"). It's obviously easier to express your anger to a person than it is to a company or an organization, but that's what protests, boycotts, and letter-writing campaigns are for!

## WHAT DOES ANGER FEEL LIKE?

This might seem like a ridiculous question because we all know what it's like to feel furious; your heart races, you can feel the blood rising to your face, and your focus on the thing that's angering you is sharp and all-encompassing. But why do we feel this way? Anger triggers the fight response of the fight or flight instinct. Adrenaline is released into your bloodstream, and you feel motivated to act to correct a wrong and, possibly, to strike back. Your heart rate increases, your blood pressure can increase, and so can your breathing. If you're frequently angry, it can damage your heart health, cause high blood pressure and inadequate sleep, depress your immune system, and give you digestive problems. [1]

## WHAT CAUSES ANGER?

Anger, an emotion that we can experience in complicated ways, has a very simple cause. Anger happens **when you have an expectation of a person, group or entity that isn't met**. It also happens when someone does something that you didn't expect and that has a negative effect on you. Certainly, there are times that you experience anger because a situation is different from what you expected, such as experiencing a flat tire on a busy freeway; however, usually the experience of anger is embedded in interpersonal relationships. Interpersonal processes are complex social interactions that involve thoughts, values, beliefs, motivations, and behaviors. [2] What makes anger, unlike the other stress emotions, a complex emotion to deal with is that it commonly involves other people (what their values and beliefs are, your beliefs about yourself and others, including what you think is right or wrong). To deal with anger effectively, it is important to be assertive in expressing both your expectations and anger in a constructive manner. Although it seems counterintuitive, people who are really uncomfortable being assertive can overreact when they're angry, lose control, and become extraordinarily explosive and unpleasant when expressing their anger.

## TYPES OF ANGER

There are two types of anger: situational and chronic. Situational anger lasts for short periods of time and goes away when you constructively express it. A beneficial byproduct of situational anger is that it can stimulate you to act – it can empower you to assert yourself. Situational anger, unlike chronic anger, can be energizing and constructive.

| TYPES OF ANGER | |
| --- | --- |
| **SITUATIONAL ANGER** | **CHRONIC ANGER** |
| • Short lived<br>• Expressed constructively<br>• Can be energizing | • Lasts for weeks/months/years<br>• Not expressed or not expressed constructively<br>• Doesn't feel good, debilitating |

## SITUATIONAL ANGER AND EMPOWERMENT

You can use your anger to positively shape your relationships with family, friends, and coworkers. To positively shape your relationships with others, it is important that you are able to experience a sense of personal power. *Being empowered means having the ability to act or influence.* Learning to be assertive is an empowering skill. The following content on assertiveness is adapted from Elizabeth Scott.[3,4]

### ASSERTIVENESS

**Assertiveness** is an important communication skill that is characterized by clearly and confidently conveying your ideas, desires, needs, and rights while still respecting the other person's rights and boundaries. Assertive messages are open and honest and typically focused on a *win-win* as the desired outcome.

Assertiveness differs from aggressive communications (and its reverse, passive communications). Aggressive communications are conveyed in an intimidating, demeaning, or threatening manner without respect for the other per son. Often that kind of aggression is motivated by a *win-lose* intent. Sometimes aggressive communications are so amplified, they're actually abusive. Passive communications that are still aggressive in their intent include silence or communicating messages in an intentionally unclear way.

## ASSERTIVENESS AS AN IMPORTANT SKILL IN RELATIONSHIPS

Many people find it difficult to be open and honest in communicating needs and desires or to give meaningful feedback due to a fear of alienating or hurting others. In reality, *not* asserting your thoughts, feelings, emotions, needs, or desires is harmful to others as it leads to unclear expectations and relationship problems both at work and at home.

The ability to be assertive is definitely related to self-esteem. When you don't feel good about yourself and don't have a sense of competence and confidence, it is very difficult to express your ideas, desires, needs, and rights openly and in a constructive manner.

## HERE ARE SOME EXAMPLES OF AGGRESSIVE, PASSIVE, AND ASSERTIVE COMMUNICATIONS

**Standing in line** — You're in line to buy movie theater tickets or at the cafeteria and someone cuts in line in front of you.

| AGGRESSIVE RESPONSE | "Hey, jerk who do you think you are!?" |
|---|---|
| PASSIVE RESPONSE | Say nothing but fume inside. |
| ASSERTIVE RESPONSE | "Excuse me, but we are in line here — it would be nice for you to take your place at the end of the line." |

**Unwelcome interruption at the office** — You're in your office and a coworker comes in and wants to tell you about an uncomfortable interaction they had with the administrator. It's 2:00 p.m., and you really don't have time to talk because you have a report due by 8:00 a.m. and you're leaving at 4:00 p.m. to pick up your child from daycare.

| AGGRESSIVE RESPONSE | "Get over it – go find someone else who cares!" |
|---|---|
| PASSIVE RESPONSE | Say nothing and talk as long as the person stays – giving up your own need to finish the report, which will then have an impact on your family/children when you have to spend time in the evening doing the report. |
| ASSERTIVE RESPONSE | "Sounds like you're having a difficult time – I am sorry I don't have the time to talk about it now – I have to get this report done by 4:00 . . . can we talk tomorrow?" |

**Expressing your idea** - You're in an important meeting that will influence how your department operates, and the chair of the meeting is incorrectly assuming that your department does not play a role in the change.

| AGGRESSIVE RESPONSE | "Well this is just like always – people like you go around making changes without knowing what you're talking about or having any idea of the unintended damage it will do to an essential function of the company. Frankly, I don't know how you got to the position you're in!" |
|---|---|
| PASSIVE RESPONSE | Say nothing but fume inside, creating a negative environment for your department. The company suffers. |

| | |
|---|---|
| **ASSERTIVE RESPONSE** | "I think the desired change has merit, and I would like to make it clear that the ____ Department plays an important role in that activity by _____. If the change is made as anticipated, without consideration of _____, it will result in _____ which will create a barrier to the company's goal to _____. Perhaps we could talk further about how to make the change in a way that it wouldn't require _____." |

**Saying no** – A co-worker, friend, or family member asks you to do something that you do not want to do and don't have time to do.

| | |
|---|---|
| **AGGRESSIVE RESPONSE** | "I can't believe that you're asking me that – don't you know I'm busy. Do you think you are the center of the universe?" |
| **PASSIVE RESPONSE** | Say nothing but fume inside and get mad at the person for asking you to do this. |
| **ASSERTIVE RESPONSE** | "I would love to do that for you; however, I'm just overloaded right now, and it's not possible for me to commit time/effort to something else . . . is there any chance that the task could be postponed until next month, or is there one small part of the task that would take about 15 or 30 minutes?" |

## HOW CAN YOU BECOME MORE ASSERTIVE?

It's helpful to strive for a win-win in difficult situations – where both people are understood and where both can get their needs met. It's dangerous, and generally wrong, to assume that you know the motives of others. Remember, it's easier to think negatively rather than positively, so when you assume what others motives are, you are more likely to assume that they are negative. You could be absolutely wrong in assuming a negative motive. Remind yourself to listen intently and to ask questions to help you understand the other person's point of view. Here are some principles to remember that should be helpful.

## TIPS ON BEING MORE ASSERTIVE

**1. Use 'I' statements. When you start off by saying, *you*, it can feel to the other person, and to you, as though you are being judgmental or attacking. Focus on the facts, your expectations or understandings, and name the emotion you are feeling.**

EXAMPLE 1: A colleague, Mark, is habitually late for meetings and appointments with you.

| AGGRESSIVE RESPONSE | "You're so rude!" or "You're always late." |
|---|---|
| ASSERTIVE RESPONSE | "Mark, our meeting was supposed to start at 9:00 a.m.; it's now 9:20. I expected that you would be here on time as you promised . . . as you know we could not proceed without your deliverables as our discussion was dependent on the results of your work, which was to be presented at the beginning of the meeting." |

EXAMPLE 2: You have a meeting scheduled with the same colleague the next week for 3:00 p.m.

| AGGRESSIVE RESPONSE | "I can't believe it – I can never count on you being on time – you are so inconsiderate!" |
|---|---|

| ASSERTIVE RESPONSE | "Tom, our appointment was for 3:00 p.m., It is now 3:25, and I have to leave at 4:00 p.m. to pick up my son from daycare – I'm really not happy because I expected that you would be on time so that we could get our work done . . . we really need to talk about your habit of not being on time. But that needs to wait until later – right now the priority is our work task. How do you propose that the work get completed?" |
|---|---|

## 2. State what the person did and, then, how you felt in response to what was done.

**"When you** [other person's behavior]**, I feel** [your feelings]**."**

When used with factual statements, rather than judgments or labels, this formula provides a direct, non-attacking, more responsible way of letting people know how their behavior affects you. For example:

"When you yell, I feel attacked."

**A more advanced variation of this blueprint includes the results of their behavior (again, put into factual terms), and looks like this:**

**"When you** [other person's behavior]**, then** [results of the behavior]**, and I feel** [how you feel]**."**

EXAMPLES:

| "When you arrive late, I have to wait, and I feel frustrated." |
|---|
| "When you tell the children they can do something that I've already forbidden, some of my authority as a parent is taken away, and I feel undermined." |

**Empower yourself.** Use situational anger to empower yourself to collect data and act to change what is changeable – enhance *your* Power!

Let me share one of my favorite examples of how someone enhanced her power in this way. Florence Nightingale is an extraordinary hero for nurses because she used her anger to create opportunities for nurses to practice and improve healthcare in general. She didn't let appalling conditions in the London hospitals, or a lack of respect by physicians at Barrack Hospital in Scutari, Turkey stop her. She used her anger to energize her action. In fact, she took advantage of every opportunity to help the physicians to see that the patients desperately needed nursing care. She worked hard to obtain the supplies needed to provide injured soldiers with adequate nutrition, fresh air, and clean beds. The men at Scutari referred to her ability to get things done as "Nightingale power".[5] The important thing about Nightingale's anger is that, **although it was frequent, her anger was situational, data driven, and about matters that were changeable. She, then, used the results of her anger to effect the change that was so sorely needed.**

**Use situational anger to act.** A realistic expectation is one that has a reasonable chance of being met. There are three elements that must exist for an expectation of another person to be realistic. (See "Criteria for Realistic Expectation" on page 177.)

## DEALING EFFECTIVELY WITH SITUATIONAL ANGER

When you experience situational anger, use the following guide to help you relate to the other person in terms of the clarity of the expectation, the individual's capability, and willingness.

**Clearly communicate the expectation.** If the expectation has been clearly communicated, and you believe the person has the ability to meet the expectation, then it is important to communicate your feeling. Constructive expression of anger is characterized by:

1) Owning it – using 'I' statements.
2) Identifying the expectation that was not met
3) Communicating a caring concern for the other person
4) Discussing the circumstances surrounding the expectation to determine if the person really is capable and/or is willing to do what you expect – is there something that can be done to get X to happen?

## CRITERIA FOR REALISTIC EXPECTATION

1. EXPECTATION WAS CLEARLY COMMUNICATED
2. PERSON HAS THE CAPABILITY TO MEET EXPECTATION
3. PERSON IS WILLING TO DO WHAT IS REQUESTED

It is often difficult for people to communicate their irritation or anger because they're apprehensive that saying how they feel out loud may have negative consequences. More often than not, if there are negative consequences from the expression of anger, it is because the communication had a blaming or judging tone ("It's your fault that I'm angry.") or the anger was expressed with an intent to hurt or harm the other person ("I should know that you're not capable of caring about other people.")

On the other hand, anger can be expressed constructively by pausing to think through how to say what your expectation was and that it wasn't met. However, if you choose not to communicate your anger, then it is important let go of the expectation because ruminating about it will only create resentment and intensify your anger. One of the major underlying reasons we struggle with this issue of expectations of others is that humans participate in a phenomenon known as *automatic knowing* or mind reading where you assume that the other person can read your mind or knows what you want.[7].

EXAMPLE:

> It's like a spouse who knows that she is going to be late for dinner tomorrow night because she has a business meeting. She tells her husband, "Honey, I'm going to be late — tomorrow night – 8:30 or 9:00 p.m." He says, "Fine." Throughout the next day, she has fleeting thoughts that certainly he'll know to prepare dinner for himself and the children. She comes home, finds him sitting in the same chair, and nothing has been done. She gets angry and expresses her anger. He replies that he didn't know that's what she expected – which typically makes her even angrier because: he should have known. As human beings who function daily on automatic pilot, we rely on patterns of behavior, not exceptions to the rule. So, if she typically fixes dinner and all she said was, "I'm going to be late," the message he received was that dinner will be late!

**Facilitate another's capability.** To be capable, a person must have the necessary knowledge, skill, and resources (material, time, social support) to carry out a desired action, and the situation must enable the action. To enhance capability means to *get out of the way* or remove blocks to a person taking a desired action. *Getting out of the way* might mean giving someone the authority to act — not just the responsibility for an action. It might also mean removing barriers to action, such as replacing a computer that doesn't work, assuring the availability of resources like an assistant in a busy office, making sure the ingredients for a sandwich are in the house. It also means taking time to understand the other person's perspective and what they need to carry out the action. Sometimes, assessing capability simply requires asking, "Is this something that you think is doable at this time, or is there anything you need to be able to make this happen?" At other times, the determination of capability requires observation over time while being clear about expectations.

**CHRONIC ANGER IS CAUSED BY HOLDING ONTO AN EXPECTATION THAT IS NOT REALISTIC!**

**Enhance willingness.** The concept of willingness, and how to encourage it in others, is one of the more challenging parts of creating realistic expectations. It is particularly difficult to influence someone to be willing to engage with what you need and expect when you don't have authority over that person. When you have authority, as a parent or a supervisor, you have the power to influence a child or an employee's willingness to perform a task or activity. When you don't have authority, you can go to decision makers, as Florence Nightingale did, armed with data. Decision makers are often hard-pressed to ignore data. If you're having a problem where you work, you can try this with your supervisor. Collect data on issues you're concerned about and present it, along with suggestions on how to refine or enhance the delivery of services or products. You can also do this at home. Collect and present data that can be discussed as a family – for example, data on spending habits. It is important to remember that, although there might be some things you can do to influence another's willingness, *it is not possible to control other people*. You can give it a shot, but if your efforts don't result in a change – let it go! If you don't, your anger will be exacerbated and undoubtedly lead to less-than-desirable consequences.

A realistic expectation is one that has a
reasonable chance of being met!

## CHRONIC ANGER

Every change that alters our role responsibilities (what we expect from each other and how we interact with each other) becomes fertile territory for chronic anger. Chronic anger is a particularly debilitating emotion that can cause uncomfortable physical symptoms, including fatigue, depression, a decrease in productivity, hostility at work, and burnout.[7.8]

Chronic anger robs us of our energy and creativity[9] and is contagious — like misery, it loves company. It's fairly common to hear employees in a breakroom sharing their irritation and anger about someone or something at work. In an unfortunate way, it's comforting to interact with people who share the anger. Unfortunately, though (surprise!), that kind of commiseration winds up stoking the flames of anger and all the negative symptoms that come with it. Sharing irritation or anger with others is really only helpful when you can get constructive feedback on how to effectively address the problematic situation.

Sadly, when we experience chronic anger it deprives us of making meaningful contributions or shaping a new reality for ourselves and others. By learning how to prevent and eliminate chronic anger, you can develop better relationships characterized by mutual understanding and respect.

**Chronic anger is caused by holding onto an expectation that is unrealistic.** Your current *demand load* might be stretching resources and making it difficult for you to meet family role responsibilities or expectations at work. You expect to have the finances to meet basic needs, the help of others when needed, a comfortable workload that permits you, and others, to perform your jobs well, and a boss who acknowledges your contributions and provides support when needed.[10] But these ideal situations frequently are not reality.

Again, the three criteria that must be met for an expectation to be realistic are:

1) The expectation has been clearly communicated.

2) The person, organization, or company has the resources (i.e., capability, knowledge, time, material resources) to meet the expectation.

3) The person, organization, or company is willing to do what is expected. [11]

Why do we hold onto unrealistic expectations? Because we believe we have a right to expect them.[12] You do have rights: the right to be treated respectfully, the right to have grievances heard, the right to be cared about, etc. However, **having a right to expect something doesn't mean that the expectation will be met**. When your rights are not honored, when your sense of right has been ignored – it's an emotionally charged situation.

Unfortunately, we raise young people to have unrealistic expectations by giving them trophies just for showing up regardless of ability. Millennials have been vulnerable to chronic anger because many expected to go to college, graduate, get a good paying job, and become independent – they did not expect to move back in with their parents. In fact, many grew up expecting economic independence to be easy to achieve, so, when the country experienced a recession and lost over 850,000 jobs, it was an unexpected and devastating situation for many.

## PREVENTING CHRONIC ANGER

To prevent chronic anger in relationships ask yourself, *was my expectation realistic? Did I communicate my expectation clearly? Did I verify that the situation would enable him/her to do what was expected? Did I inquire about willingness to do it?* It is also important for you to manage your own expectations in social situations and at work given your knowledge of the organization's dynamics and developmental phase. For example, several years ago I had the pleasure of meeting a young registered nurse who had been practicing as a staff nurse since 1994. I was conducting a workshop on conquering stress in the workplace, and she was on a panel of nurses who shared how they were coping with all of the turmoil in nursing practice. Her hospital was in the final phases of implementing the latest re-engineering of nursing care delivery. She was incredibly upbeat and positive. A nurse in the audience said, "Aren't you tired of all of the changes? Don't you get stressed out or angry?"

The nurse on the panel said:

*Since I've been in practice for five years, change is all I've known. This is my third redesign of how we deliver nursing care. I know the leadership at my hospital is doing the best they can to cut costs so that we can stay in the business of taking care of sick people. They frequently seek our input on how we can deliver the best care with fewer resources. We have great feedback systems, so, when something isn't working, we try to fix it. It's a challenge every day, but I don't experience anger about it.* **I think I'm advantaged, because all I've known is change. I expect it! I love what I do!**

Expecting change in the workplace gives you an upfront advantage in preventing chronic anger because the vast majority of businesses, whether in healthcare or business sectors, are continuously focused on cost cutting and process improvements.

## ALLEVIATING CHRONIC ANGER

When one or more of the criteria for a realistic expectation are not met, the stage is set for chronic anger. As previously noted, chronic anger is debilitating. **If you are prone to experience chronic anger, ask yourself this question,** *Who is hurt by the anger I experience?* Ninety percent of the time (excluding when people abuse others or commit crimes out of anger), it's you not the other person, organization, or company who is hurt by the anger. A few years ago, on the *Oprah* show, there was a segment on chronic anger and the untoward psychological and physical effects it has on the person experiencing it. A powerful point was made: *"Allowing yourself to experience chronic anger is like you drinking poison and hoping it harms the other person!"*

> **ALLOWING YOURSELF TO EXPERIENCE CHRONIC ANGER IS LIKE YOU DRINKING THE POISON AND HOPING IT HARMS THE OTHER PERSON!**

When chronic anger is experienced, the cure is to *let go of the expectation*, that is, stop expecting it. Easier said than done? Yes. However, for each of the common beliefs that make it difficult to let go, there is a strategy that will help. The next section reviews each of these.

## LETTING GO

Letting go can be difficult because, after all, you believe you have a right to expect what you are not receiving! Right? Well, in some instances that might be true (as would be the case in situations of verbal or physical abuse), but, even in these instances, the important action to take is to modify your situation by leaving it, thereby letting go. Rather than staying to change the situation, leaving is one of the strongest examples of letting go. Letting go is easier when you understand the dynamics that keep you holding on. Let us look at a few of these.

*If I let go, it means they win and I lose!* A common belief that makes letting go difficult is the belief that if you let go, the other person wins! Think about it – there is *no* winner here - it's just you suffering. I doubt very much that the other person is suffering – in fact, the other person might not even know that you are experiencing chronic anger. Or, if the other person

> **IT'S YOUR CHOICE TO CONTINUE TO EXPERIENCE ANGER!**

knows you're angry all of the time, it seemingly makes no difference to them. Perhaps some people who experience chronic anger *like* to suffer or play the martyr, but there is no pay-off for such experiences. In fact, if the person who experiences chronic anger continually expresses the anger to people not involved in the situation, pretty soon it creates wear and tear on others. And, they may feel like they cannot share with you how old the complaining is getting or that it is unpleasant to be around.

*Hope Isn't Always The Answer.* It's fairly common for people to experience chronic anger at home or work about what other people do or don't do. As mentioned earlier, one of the most helpful strategies here for letting go is to **start expecting the person to do what you *know* they are going to do (or not do).** One of the worst emotions that you can have in this type of a situation is *hope*. *I hope that tomorrow will be different . . . that Scott will do his job and not leave some of it for me to do.* Hope keeps you hanging onto expectations. If you've discussed the situation with the person, and you have no authority over the consequences, as well as ample experience with the situation not changing then, **expect it not to be different tomorrow.** There might be work that you still need to do, that is not part of your job, and you can plan for this. But, you won't suffer because of it. It is your *choice* to continue to experience the anger. Sure, you might work harder and get more done than the other person, but getting angry about it doesn't change the situation – you just suffer. In a work situation, it may be possible *not* to do the work the other person left undone (if it isn't necessary for your work or won't cause harm) and, then, hope that the unfinished work will have negative consequences for the other person.

With teenagers who refuse to keep their bedroom straight and clean, it's your choice to experience chronic anger or to just let go and shut the door! I would only get concerned in this situation if critters start multiplying in the bedroom, but, then, I would just call the exterminator! If you let go, and stop expecting something, you have the opportunity to be pleasantly surprised should it ever happen!

It's your choice to get angry when your husband doesn't pick up his dirty clothes from the bedroom floor. I worked with a grieving widow several years ago. As Nancy was reminiscing about her husband, she said to me:

*You know I frequently got angry with him about some things now that seem so insignificant – like leaving his dirty socks and pants on the floor and not putting them in the laundry basket. Today, I would give anything to come home and find his dirty clothes on the bedroom floor. Losing Ted really puts into perspective what's important and what isn't!*

**I expect them to treat me with respect — I expect that from any human being!** Well, this is an interesting irrational belief. Many of us have ample experience with people who do *not* have the capacity to respect others or to demonstrate respect for others. Respect is often defined differently by each person. What respect looks like to you may be quite different from what it looks like to the other person. I learned many years ago that, to help eliminate this expectation, it can be helpful to visualize the other person as something different from what you actually see. For example, you might visualize the person as an animal that does not have human potential. Pick an animal that you think is cute/funny/pleasant to be around, such as a koala. Visualize the person's body as the animal that you have selected and silently ask yourself, *what can I expect from a koala?* Using this strategy helped me let go of unrealistic expectations of an administrator I reported to early in my career. Amazingly, communication between the other person and me actually improved because I stopped expecting her to be or do something that she wasn't or couldn't.

The belief that everyone should treat you with respect is the foundation for a lot of the road rage experienced today. *People should have learned how to be courteous to others and respect the rights of others on the road . . . isn't that taught in driver's education?* Each of us certainly has ample experience with the fact that the belief is false. I know people who experience anger every time they drive. In fact, they talk with – or yell/cuss at – other drivers as if the other drivers can hear what they are saying!!?? I've modified my expectations by being very clear that, every time I get in my car to drive, what I'm really doing is going to a wild kingdom – there are lots of cute and entertaining animals out there that are also totally unpredictable. So, I expect strange maneuvers and accept that many of the zoo residents can't read road signs!

***If they don't do what I expect, it means there's an absence of love or care.*** I have found that this irrational belief occurs all too often in marriages. In part because of this unfortunate belief, premarital counseling has come into vogue. Thank goodness. When people commit to each other in a relationship, it's critical that each understands that what happens before the marriage will likely continue to happen after the marriage.

I recall one client of mine in the late 1980s. She was referred to me by a physician because of a number of abdominal symptoms that had no discernible pathology, and he thought that it might be stress-related – a very astute physician he was! Carol was in her late 20s. She had been married to Stan for three years prior to their divorce. It was about 10 months after the divorce when I first met with her. Her primary stress emotions were chronic anger and unjustified guilt, which both lingered since the divorce. Carol continuously relived the circumstances in which she experienced anger with Stan where she felt guilty that she was not "a good enough wife" for him to do what she expected. As it turns out, her chronic anger with Stan stemmed from minor expectations, e.g. *he should know how to squeeze the toothpaste tube properly or to put the toilet seat down when he leaves the bathroom!* At the time we met, Carol had become aware of the fact that her expectations were, in essence, about little things that just drove her up a wall. That realization did not stop her from ruminating about all of the things that she used to get angry about. It did enhance the guilt that she experienced because she made such a big deal out of everything. (This is also a good example of unjustified guilt because she truly didn't know any better at the time – she can, however, learn from the experience.)

To help Carol learn from her experience and how to let go, we focused on the chronic anger situation with the tube of toothpaste. I helped her imagine a typical situation in which she experienced anger with Stan over the toothpaste tube. (*By the way, I asked her what 'properly' meant to her because I didn't grow up in a household where I learned the 'proper' way to squeeze a toothpaste tube – we just squeezed it. 'Proper' to Carol included 3 criteria: Squeeze from the* bottom, *flatten the tube and then roll it up. Well – talk about an unreasonable assumption!*) At any rate, I helped her remember a typical situation where she was angry with Stan. This is how she described the morning situation. They lived in a two-bedroom apartment with one bath. Stan would get up first in the morning, do what he needed to do in the bathroom to get ready for work, and be sitting in the kitchen drinking a cup of coffee. Carol would walk into the bathroom and see the tube of toothpaste lying on the side of the sink with a big gouge in the middle of it. Here is her internal dialogue:

> *I don't know how many times I need to tell him. I've shown him how it should be done and asked a thousand times [probably an exaggeration] that he do it properly. I mean how much effort can it take to do it properly. He just doesn't seem to care. I even bought him that little metal clip to help with flattening and rolling. When I think of all the things that I do for him . . . [a substantial pause] . . . . I don't know why I bother! He must not love me because, if he did, he would do this little thing.* **Ouch!** *[An interesting point – in our internal dialogue we answer the questions we ask ourselves.]*

Every morning, Carol suffered while Stan (who by the way, treated her quite nicely, on the whole) went about his usual morning routine. It is important to note that how we do many things have become *habits*, including how we squeeze a toothpaste tube, and habits are hard to break. I don't know what Stan was thinking. Maybe he thought that how he squeezed the toothpaste tube couldn't be that important. Maybe he got tired of her nagging about it and just tuned her out – whatever he thought, squeezing the toothpaste tube never rose to the top of his priority list in terms of behavior change. I don't know if Stan loved her or not, and it's likely that Stan contributed to difficulties in their relationship in some way, but I am confident that her chronic anger probably didn't help the relationship.

What Carol learned from our work together was how powerful our internal dialogue is and to **let go by expecting what you know will happen to happen rather than hoping it will change.** And, if it's so important for something to be done a certain way (the tube to be squeezed properly), then she should do it herself. Carol learned that having perspective on what is and isn't important in a relationship will help her in future relationships. After alleviating her ruminating chronic anger, working on alleviating her guilt feelings (by learning to forgive herself), and being confident that the marriage provided her an opportunity to learn an important relationship skill, her gastrointestinal symptoms disappeared. It's fascinating to me how common it is for women who experience chronic guilt to experience gastrointestinal symptoms. Perhaps there is a phenomenon here that should be named and studied, something like regret or remorse stomach.

*He abused or harmed me, and he should suffer more!* Letting go in the case of abuse or harm is even more difficult because it involves forgiving the other person or people. Hanging onto chronic anger in the case of harm is particularly devastating because the person experiencing the anger will often experience somatic symptoms or physical discomforts or a debilitating psychological illness. Forgiving doesn't mean forgetting. Luskin identifies what forgiveness is *not*:

- Condoning unkindness,
- Forgetting that something painful has happened,
- Excusing poor behavior,
- Denying or minimizing hurt, or
- Reconciling with the offender.[13]

Luskin notes that just because someone hurt you does not mean you have to suffer indefinitely.

As Luskin asserts, forgiveness is a choice – it doesn't change the past, it changes the present and how you feel now and in the future. Once you realize that continuing to experience the anger (and all of the accompanying discomforts) causes suffering, it helps the letting go process in the case of harm. Furthermore, continuing to experience anger is *relinquishing control of your emotions* to that person who caused the harm.

I have worked with clients who have experienced harms such as sexual abuse, being shot by a robber, being fired from a job so that a pension didn't have to be paid, being seriously injured as a result of a car accident caused by a drunk driver, and losing a husband due to medical malpractice. In all of these instances, the chronic anger experienced by these individuals was, in itself, debilitating and was only cured by learning how to forgive the other person.

It is important to note that when you let go of an expectation, you don't need to disclose to the other person that you have stopped expecting something or that you have forgiven them — it just needs to occur in your internal dialogue. Definitely, in the case of forgiveness, your letting go needs to be truly felt in your heart.

## TIPS TO DEAL EFFECTIVELY WITH SITUATIONAL AND CHRONIC ANGER

**To effectively deal with interpersonal situational anger:**

1. Clearly communicate the expectation that wasn't met.

2. Calmly communicate the emotion you experienced, such as irritation, annoyance, or anger using 'I' statements ("When I saw that X was not done, I experienced anger.")

3. Ask if the expectation was realistic/doable.

4. Ask if something happened that made it difficult to accomplish.

5. Ask if it is reasonable for you to expect it in the future.

**To effectively prevent interpersonal chronic anger, ask yourself:**

1. Have I clearly communicated the expectation?

2. Have I checked with the person to validate that it is doable?

3. Have I checked with the person that he/she is willing?

4. Have I verified that he/she has everything needed to meet the expectation?

> **WHEN YOU FEEL THAT SOMEONE IS ANGRY WITH YOU, ASK THE PERSON, "WHAT DID YOU EXPECT THAT DIDN'T HAPPEN?"** FOCUS THE CONVERSATION ON IF THE EXPECTATION WAS COMMUNICATED CLEARLY, WAS DOABLE, AND WHETHER OR NOT YOU ARE WILLING.

**To alleviate chronic anger:**

1. First, recognize it!

2. Let go of the expectation – STOP expecting it! (Beware of hope keeping you hanging on!)

3. Expect what you know will likely happen.

## SUMMARY

While situational anger can be empowering, chronic anger is commonly harmful to your health and your relationships. The cause of anger, whether situational or chronic, is that you had an expectation that was not met. Expectations can be the bane of our existence if they are not communicated clearly and if your expectation is not realistic. The skill of communicating your expectations clearly will serve you well both in relationships and at work.

The next chapter focuses on frustration, which although not an emotion, provides fertile ground to experience any one of the stress emotions.

# CHAPTER 9

# CONQUERING
# FRUSTRATION

They conquer who believe they can.

— RALPH WALDO EMERSON

We've all experienced frustration, but why is it a separate chapter apart from anger? Frustration is closely related to anger, as explained below, but by itself is not an emotion. Many assert that frustration is an emotion because it often results in some level of anger, from irritation to rage. Frustration, however, is a specific perception or psychological state of mind that is often a precursor to anger and can trigger anxiety and guilt. You can both prevent and eliminate frustration if you follow the principles in this chapter. Like the principles on preventing stress emotions discussed in previous chapters, it's not rocket science, but it does take knowledge, self-awareness, and effort.

## WHAT IS FRUSTRATION?

We all know what frustration feels like, but how often are we asked to define it? I'm sure your answer is the same as mine, rarely to never. But, understanding what frustration is, of course, the key to defeating it. Frustration is a mental recognition that something internal or external is getting in the way of accomplishing a task or goal. In fact, the definition of the verb *to frustrate* is exactly that: to prevent an individual or group from accomplishing a goal. You know when you go to the ATM and, no matter what you do, the machine keeps spitting your card out at you, and you can't access your cash? That machine is blocking your efforts to get your money, which results in frustration, which, in turn, can trigger some level of anger. Frustration is closely related to anger because, like anger, it results from an expectation not being met. A goal is a type of expectation. You expect to accomplish what you set out to accomplish. When your expectation isn't met, some level of anger, from irritation to rage, is often triggered. When a block prevents you from doing something or achieving a goal, it can trigger guilt. When a block prevents you from securing your safety, it can trigger anxiety. Because frustration is closely related to anger, anxiety and guilt, it is easy to assume that it is an emotion.

## WHAT DOES FRUSTRATION FEEL LIKE?

Using an unscientific description, frustration feels like your head is in a tizzy; it is vexing, unsettling, or aggravating. Intense frustration can feel like your head is going to blow off. You know when you've tried to fix a paper jam in a printer for the seventh time and you still can't get your report (due in five minutes) printed and you find yourself cursing and hitting the machine with your balled-up fists? That is frustration triggering anger. Again, the stress emotions that frustration can give rise to are anger, anxiety, guilt, and, if long lasting, perhaps even situational depression. Frustration is not fun.

## WHAT CAUSES FRUSTRATION?

Simply put, you become frustrated when you have a goal and something or someone prevents you from accomplishing it. Again, it is an expectation not met. The blocks to your goal can be internal or external. Internal blocks include unclear goals, impatience, not breaking goals down into doable steps, lack of confidence, a lack of knowledge/information, a lack of skill or competence, internal conflict (the goal is in conflict with something else you want to be or accomplish), and even fear of accomplishment, which can occur when accomplishing a goal might change others' expectations of you – they might expect even more of you.

External blocks include physical roadblocks, lack of a resource (such as money), a bus that doesn't arrive on time, a printer that isn't working, or people/rules/regulations preventing actions. Frustration can also happen when you try to set goals for others. When you set a goal for your family, your company, your friends, or a club, it gets more complicated with multiple people in the equation. Even if you set a goal for another person or a group, and all the circumstances are right, you can still experience enormous frustration if even one member of the group doesn't get on board with your plan. If you don't have unanimous buy-in, you're headed straight for the agonies of frustration!

Let me make the issue of frustration a little more vivid by providing you with typical things you might hear from a frustrated person (including yourself)!

*It's been a wild day and, once again, I'm feeling frustrated. There's always something getting in my way. Since October of last year,*

*I've wanted to go back to school, and now October has rolled around again and nothing has changed; I'm still not in school, work is hectic, and home life is frenzied.*

*One of my New Year's resolutions was to lose twenty pounds. It's the end of January, and, despite working really hard to watch what I eat and to exercise, I've only lost four pounds in 30 days. I'm ready to give up!*

**Preventing and Eliminating Frustration.** If you want to keep frustration at bay, you have to remember that you REAP what you sow. REAP is an acronym I use to remind myself, and my clients, of the set of principles that help you to deal effectively with, or avoid, frustration.[2] The principles are easy to understand but can be difficult to consistently implement, primarily because they take a little time to get used to and use. Always remember that *impatience is not your friend!* Here are the REAP principles.

## R STANDS FOR *REALISTIC*

The goals you set must be realistic, which means *achievable*. A goal must be *clear* to be achievable. You must know specifically what it is you want to accomplish. Setting an unclear goal such as, *I want to have more money,* is stress-inducing because it's not clear enough. Your goal should specify exactly what outcome you'd like, the time-frame you'd need to accomplish it, and tasks or strategies to accomplish the goal.

A specific and realistic goal would be, *I want to save $200 a month. I'll do that by not buying a venti coffee every morning at Starbucks and taking my lunch to work.* By identifying clear goals, and the corresponding actions to reach those goals, you'll bypass the frustration of an unclear goal like, *I want to have more money.*

It's true that it can be difficult to know if your goal is realistic before you set out to accomplish it. With that said, often what makes a goal unrealistic is the amount of time you give yourself to accomplish it. If you're not sure that a goal is achievable for you, seek some feedback from another person who knows you or has achieved the same or similar goal. Don't pick a naysayer, pick someone you can trust and can perhaps even mentor you as you work to accomplish your goal. There is support available to help you accomplish your goals, such as mentors identified through the Small Business Administration or academic counselors, or even groups to help you overcome an addiction.

Even when a goal *is* realistic, things can get in the way of achieving it — some blocks are external, and others you personally generate. A common external block includes insufficient resources like time and money. It's important to recognize that both of these things can be changed or eliminated by how you spend your time and money. If you do not have time to cook dinner for your family, purchase a prepared dinner at the grocery store or plan ahead by making double and freezing it. Be creative. Generate several alternative ways to accomplish your goal.

Other external blocks are difficult or not possible to change. They include other people and organizational culture that is too ingrained or big for you to change on your own. However, many times, when you cannot change the external obstacle to your goal, you can find ways to go around or avoid the block. For example, if the organization you're working in does not support you taking time off to earn a degree or take classes to become certified in your discipline, you can take courses online and do your course work at night and on the weekends. The incredible advantage of today's technology is that there are numerous ways for you to accomplish personal goals in non-traditional ways.

One of the most common internal blocks to attaining a goal is a negative view of possibilities due to a lack of information. We often imagine blocks that really aren't there or that more information could solve. It was fairly common for me to hear someone say, "I'd really like to become a nurse, but I'm sure I can't afford it." When you assume something is true without checking, the possible can become impossible. When I heard that statement, I would give the person the phone number for a student advisor at the school of nursing. Invariably, when the person followed through and made an appointment, he or she found that there are many scholarships available. Don't let insufficient information or invalid conclusions block you from something you want to accomplish!

Not managing your time well is also a common internally-generated block. Time management not only requires that you determine the best use of your time to accomplish a goal but also that you find ways to work smarter.

Think about a typical day in your life. How much of your time is eaten up by demands that are non-essential or irrelevant to your goals? Is it really necessary to clean your house thoroughly every Saturday? Is it really necessary that you be on so many committees? Is it essential that you say yes to every request? Stop attending to those demands that aren't important to your goals.

## E STANDS FOR *EFFORT*

Nobody ever accomplished a goal by sitting back and not trying. Effort requires the will to do what it takes and to be able to manage your time well. The will to do is easy to have when the goal is something that you really want to achieve.

Use your creative intellect to find quicker or easier ways to accomplish necessary tasks. In other words, be efficient. Ask yourself, *how can I get the same outcome without spending so much time on it?* How about using a foil oven bag for dinners? How about using that crockpot more often? How about buying clothes that don't require ironing? How about using lean manufacturing you've learned at work in your personal life?

## A STANDS FOR *APPORTION*

Apportion tasks required to achieve a complex goal. It is imperative that you break large, complex goals down into smaller, accomplishable tasks. If you have a goal of going back to school or getting a promotion, it helps to break what needs to be done down into identifiable tasks and set a reasonable time frame to get each task completed. This is important because, with each piece that you accomplish, you feel like you're making progress rather than feeling defeated and hopeless. I often use the example of losing weight. Many of us have set a goal of losing 20 pounds. Too often, the effort progresses as follows. You set the goal to lose twenty pounds. Then the question is when to start.

Whether you start a new way of eating and exercising on Monday or Thursday, you put forth a concerted effort for one week to reach your goal of losing twenty pounds. Then, when you get on the scale, having focused on twenty pounds, the one pound that is gone is disappointing. *I don't know why I try — I can't do it!* In reality, losing one pound/week is realistic. In fact, if your mindset was to lose one pound per week, and you saw that pound disappear on the scale, you would feel that you had accomplished your goal! You would likely be inspired to put forth the effort the next week and the weeks after that. Breaking goals down into accomplishable steps not only makes the overarching goal achievable, it enables you to feel that you are being successful from start to finish. **It prevents premature giving up.**

## P STANDS FOR *PATIENCE* AND *PERSISTENCE*

Impatience is probably the most common cause of frustration in today's world. We are all inundated with interruptions, many of them unexpected. It's important to *expect interruptions*, not get discouraged, and keep your eye on the weekly or monthly goal. Say things to yourself like, *this is not going to upset my apple cart – I'm still going to get there.*

There are also times when what you try doesn't work the first, second, or even third time around. I often think of the example set by Thomas Edison. He tried experiment after experiment in his pursuit of the incandescent light bulb. Time after time, his efforts didn't work. Edison wasn't discouraged or angry. He told a disappointed coworker that they hadn't failed because now they knew 1,000 ways that it wouldn't work, which meant they were that much closer to finding the way it *would* work.

When we're feeling like we just can't go on, it's great to remember Dr. William DeVries. He spoke frankly about his frustration in implanting the first artificial heart. In an article in the *New York Times from April 12, 1983, h*e said that if the press had not been there, he would have picked up the artificial heart, thrown it on the floor, walked out, and

> **Interesting Scale Behavior**
> Women typically weigh on Mondays and often weigh themselves dry, desiring to see the most accurate weight. That is in the morning, stark naked, after going to the bathroom, maybe even before showering so that hair has no water weight. (Also according to most women no normal person starts a diet on any day other than Monday.) Men typically don't care, weighing themselves any day, any time with all their clothes on, even shoes.

just said the patient is dead. Obviously, he didn't do that, he hung in there until he was successful.

## TIPS FOR PREVENTING FRUSTRATION

1. **R** = Set **r**ealistic goals within **r**ealistic time frames.

2. **E** = Determine what type of **e**ffort and amount of time it will take to accomplish the goal.

3. **A** = **A**pportion, or break down, large, complex goals into accomplishable steps; focus on one step at a time

4. **P** = Be **p**atient with yourself and **p**ersistent in your efforts to accomplish the goals.

## SUMMARY

The REAP principles are easy to grasp but can be a bit of a challenge to implement. Once you start really paying attention to these principles, and slowly figuring out how to incorporate them into your life, it will become a habit to think this way about goal setting and achievement. You can learn to make the REAP principles a habit by reflecting on the specifics of what's happening when you experience a block to your goal. Identify if the block is external or internal. Ask yourself:

1) Is there a way to eliminate the block or go around it?

2) Do I need more information – am I just imagining the block or is it real?

3) Do I just need to be more patient?

4) Do I need to break the goal down into more specific steps?

Successful implementation of the REAP principles will help you prevent the experience of a stress emotion when you experience a block to your goal.

# CHAPTER 10

# DEALING WITH LOSS, GRIEF AND SITUATIONAL DEPRESSION

*To spare oneself from grief at all cost can be achieved only at the price of
total detachment, which excludes the ability to experience happiness.*

— ERICH FROMM

Grief is a powerful human experience that everyone who lives
long enough to develop loving and valued attachments has to face
and deal with. As we all know, grief can be incredibly painful, even
crippling. It's essential to do what you can to address grief when it
arises since trying to avoid or bury it will only give rise to more emotional difficulty. Grief is often accompanied by situational depression
if the grief emotions are held in or not accepted as normal. The good
news is that there are ways of dealing with loss, grief, and situational
depression that can prevent devastation, while still allowing you to
experience the full range of human emotions.

## WHAT IS GRIEF?

Described in the simplest way possible, grief is a sadness that can range from feeling mildly sad to feeling profound sadness that can overwhelm you to the point of physical exhaustion. It's common to experience some level of sadness even with positive changes because you've left something you enjoyed or loved, a city, a home, a work role. Intense sadness can be mixed with disbelief, horror, heartbreak, and other emotions that can send us to our beds for relief.

Described more technically, grief is the psychological and emotional adjustment to a significant loss, which *brings about a break in continuity or disruption of patterns of doing and meaning.* Grief manifests in the experience of sadness and often involves the experience of anxiety, anger, guilt, and frustration to varying degrees.

Grief is perhaps one of the most painful human experiences. It affects people differently but is usually described, psychologically, as "experiencing a hole in the heart or soul." Emotionally, the core emotion of grief is painful sadness. It is experienced as anguish, sorrow, heartache, or heartbreak. Of course, grief feels different for different people depending on which emotions a person experiences along with the experience of loss.

## WHAT CAUSES GRIEF?

Grief is caused by the psychological recognition of a significant/ important loss. The loss can be of a person, a pet, an object, a possession, a relationship, a circumstance, or the loss of meaning or purpose. Many people don't recognize the loss of meaning or purpose as a cause for grief. Both meaning and purpose provide us with a reason for living and even a reason to get up every morning. Meaning and purpose motivate us to achieve the personal goals we set and have a profound influence on what we choose to do each day. Meaning also gives us a sense of control and contributes to our self-worth. The important role that meaning and purpose play in our lives is why people are often advised not to retire without having continued or new sense of purpose.

As noted above it's important to know that the experience of loss does not always come from a negative event. Loss can also be experienced in positive changes, such as a promotion, or a desired move to a different city. The losses occurring with positive changes can be losses in resources (e.g., convenient shopping, banking, hairdresser, physician, dentist) or in relationships (e.g., co-workers, friends, family). As we all know, change can be difficult but now you know the culprit: loss and the grief that comes with it.

## THE DYNAMICS OF GRIEF

Many people understand grief as it's been explained by Dr. Elizabeth Kubler-Ross and then picked up in popular culture. Kubler-Ross identified the five stages of grief, which you're probably already familiar with: denial, anger, bargaining, depression, and acceptance. Although Kubler-Ross's work on the experience of grief made an important contribution to our understanding of grief as a process, I, along with others, have observed some inconsistencies and important additions to Kubler-Ross's theory.

**First**, I have found that describing *denial* as *disbelief* is much more helpful. Disbelief is distinctly different from the psychiatric phenomenon of denial. I have not seen a person deny that someone or something was lost, but I have seen many who experienced disbelief. You rarely hear, "My friend *did not* move out of town!" but you will hear, "I can't believe my friend left!" It is possible that someone may experience denial in a true psychiatric sense, but, in my experience, it is usually disbelief that people experience after a loss. When my father died unexpectedly, from sudden cardiac arrest, I was out of town, and, when I was called, I thought, *how can this be?* It's not that I denied his death, but I really needed to see my father at the funeral home to make it real to me. It's hard to believe something that you haven't experienced yet is real.

**Second**, Kubler-Ross's work implies that the stages of grief occur sequentially, in the order she presented. There have been many critiques of Kubler-Ross's work. Most importantly, there is no empirical support for grief happening in the specific stages she outlines.[2,3,4] In my, and many others' experience, the grief process is not linear. This is another example of how pop culture can adopt and promote a theory that is not based on sound science.

**Third**, in working with clients who have experienced a significant loss, I've observed other important differences in their experiences from Kubler-Ross's assertions. Anxiety and sadness are very important emotional experiences not addressed in the stages theory.

I want to emphasize here that sadness is not a stress emotion. In fact, sadness is a byproduct of love or good feelings. We don't experience sadness if we lose someone or something that we have not established a bond or a loving relationship with. One of my brothers, who is an avid scratch golfer, retired early and became part owner of a private golf course. He kept busy with a new purpose managing the private club and playing golf. After selling the golf course and losing one of his eyes, he experienced a significant void. Although he was, and still is, happily married, he lost meaning and purpose. His stepdaughters gave him a labradoodle puppy, thinking that it might help but also not sure since he hated dogs. Well, he fell in love with the puppy he named Leroy. He and Leroy did a lot together every day. He had said to me on several occasions, "I hope I die before Leroy because I don't know if I could handle it if he died first." Unfortunately, he had to put Leroy down in February of 2019. It's really the first time since my father's unexpected death that I've seen him just bawl. "I lost my best friend. I never thought I could love a dog this much! I have a hole in my heart." I suggested, as did many others, that maybe he should think about getting another dog. "Absolutely not. I'm not going through this again!" Well, six months later, he and my sister-in-law went to see a new Labradoodle puppy. "I have to get another dog. It's the only way to get over Leroy – to fall in love with another dog."

Although Kubler-Ross's work made important contributions to the study of grief, I have found Peter Marris' work to be much more helpful. Peter Marris' landmark work on loss and change explains the process of grief work when there is a significant change that results in a significant loss. [5] Marris' explanation of the grief process helps us understand the important role that anxiety plays in the experience. He asserts, based on research, that as humans we rely heavily on continuity in our daily lives, on the patterns in relationships, work, play, how we function, and how we feel. These patterns are embedded in **meaning**, the reason and purpose for why we do what we do. The reliance on continuity or sameness in patterns helps us function effectively, and meaning gives us a sense of attachment and understanding. We assume, as we start each day, that the patterns so familiar to us will continue unchanged. Grief is the psychological adjustment to a significant loss that causes a break in the patterns of what we do each day, how we do it, and, often, in the meaning behind everyday actions.

It makes so much sense to understand grief as a break in continuity of familiar patterns that we rely on every day. A *break in continuity* helps to explain why grief can also be experienced even in positive changes. Although it is a positive event, it is also a change in continuity when your child leaves home for college or you accept a desired job in a different city or state you come to love. It's common to see mothers and fathers experience grief evidenced by teary-eyed goodbyes as they drop their child off at the university dorm. When an older couple decides it's time to downsize and move out of their 50-year-old family home, it's common for the couple to grieve for the home they and their children loved. It's pretty common for a person who gets promoted to a management position to experience the loss of the friendships developed as a staff employee.

All changes that include a significant disruption in continuity are experienced as loss. Some common ones include death, divorce, moving, losing a job, a major promotion, an empty nest. The stronger the meanings in existing patterns, the more intense the grief-related emotions. People commonly equate the intensity of grief with how much someone or something was loved. Although love in relationships, or for our home, or town, or for material possessions, is important, *what determines the intensity of grief is the level of disruption in patterns and meaning.*

## GRIEF WORK

Going through the grief process is work! Grief takes a toll on our emotional energy. It is common for people experiencing grief to talk about being very tired. The work of grief involves establishing continuity again, and that takes effort. It takes a lot of energy to work on establishing new patterns of being, including meaning, thinking, feeling, and behaving.

It takes time and effort for a wife who has lost her husband to establish new patterns of being. New patterns involve everything, including, but not limited to, what you do throughout the day, what you anticipate when you get home from work or grocery shopping, how you set the table, how you plan your week, who you socialize with, what you do for relaxation/vacations, how you relate to your children, how you manage finances, and how you maintain the home. It's typically more challenging to establish new patterns when the loss was sudden, as opposed to when you have time to prepare, make contingency plans, and rehearse how you will live when the loss occurs. No matter whether the loss is known in advance or is sudden, establishing new patterns is a lot of work!

While you are working on establishing new patterns and a new sense of continuity, you are also dealing with a lot of emotions, which commonly include sadness, anxiety, anger, and maybe unjustified guilt and situational depression. Again, sadness is not a stress emotion. It helps to remember that the experience of sadness is an indication that you have lost someone or something important to you. The sadness needs to be embraced. Allow yourself to experience it! It is an indication that you have lost someone or something you loved that will live forever in your heart. The sadness from the loss of a significant other never really goes away, totally. What happens is the intensity of what you feel dissipates, and the frequency of its experience lessens dramatically over time. However, every time you think of the person, there may be a twinge of sadness – that's normal!

> **"GRIEF NEVER ENDS . . . BUT IT CHANGES. IT'S A PASSAGE NOT A PLACE TO STAY. GRIEF IS NOT A SIGN OF WEAKNESS OR A LACK OF FAITH . . . IT IS THE PRICE OF LOVE."**
>
> **–UNKNOWN**

**Anxiety is a common emotion experienced in grief because the break in continuity creates many unknowns.** *Will I be able to establish new meaningful relationships? Will I be able to manage my home? Will I be able to manage my finances?* In the case of a promotion, will

*I be able to maintain relationships with my colleagues? Will I be able to be successful in my new role?* When doing grief work, it is helpful to prevent dysfunctional anxiety by anticipating positive outcomes and saying positive affirmations: *I've dealt with difficult situations in the past, I can deal with this one! This is going to be a journey. I'm going to discover what works and what doesn't. I need to be patient with myself!*

**Anger may be experienced because you certainly didn't expect to lose who or what has been lost.** Anger is particularly difficult to deal with if the loss of a loved one was due to something that was preventable or was the result of a crime. Maybe the loss of a job was due to an action that you perceive as unjust. Forgiveness is particularly important in being able to resolve or prevent chronic anger in the midst of grief work. Forgiveness isn't easy but it is a necessity if you don't want to suffer. Not forgiving results in chronic anger, which leads to you, and only you, suffering.

**Guilt may be experienced because you said something you regret saying to the person or because you didn't say something you wish you had said or because you didn't do something you think you should have done.** One thing I've learned over my adult life is that everyone always does the best they are capable of doing at the time. In fact, everyone makes the best decision possible in each situation given their state of mind, the information available, and the characteristics of a particular situation. We don't wake up every day anticipating that we're not going to see someone tomorrow or that a drunk driver is going to hit our car head on. Sure, we can adopt rules for what we do every day in our relationships, but we're not perfect. Expecting that you should be able to accurately foresee the future is an unrealistic expectation of self and results in unjustified guilt. You can forgive yourself!

**Frustration can be experienced when it takes time to establish new patterns of satisfying relationships.** Be patient. Establishing new patterns is not easy – it's what makes it work! There's a lot of trial and error. Expect that! Rarely does anything in life, that is truly meaningful, come easily. Grief work takes time. How much time it takes depends on the person and the circumstances. It's important to note here that grief unexpressed will likely take longer to work through.

I have saved one of my favorite client stories for the end, because it synthesizes much of the content in this book. Like several of my clients, Craig's stress emotions and stress-related physical illness were triggered by a loss in meaning. I had the wonderful opportunity to work with this very bright young man many years ago during one of his summer breaks from college. He was referred to me by a physician colleague/friend who was familiar with my work. He couldn't afford to pay me but wanted to compensate me in some way. I told him that I was confident that we could work together successfully, and he could pay me by writing up his experience, what he learned, and give me permission to publish his story in a book I would be writing in the future. I told him that his experience may one day help someone else.

Craig had experienced a very significant loss of his spiritual self. The specifics are not important so long as you know that the loss of his spiritual self-constituted a serious loss in meaning. The loss of his faith, which had been a critical resource for him, left him vulnerable to experience unbearable stress. Craig's story really captures the essence of the primary message in this book: *If you get in touch with your stress emotions, and change the thoughts triggering them, you change how you feel – both emotionally and physically.*

Here is Craig's story in his own words:

*It's as if an atomic bomb was detonated within the confines of your skull. Millions of fractured thoughts and emotions buzz through your head one after another. Your nerves are raw, frazzled, like a bouquet of flowers with the bulbs cut off. Your heart beats so fast, it feels as though you're having a heart attack – or have just bungee jumped out of bed. Indeed, even before you're totally awake, and before you're out of bed, these symptoms explode in your body.*

*A feeling of intense nausea followed by blurred vision plagues you as you move toward the shower. Even your hurried breakfast is disturbed because, for some strange reason, you are having trouble swallowing your food. As you leave the house to start your day, your legs feel like Jell-O, your neck aches, and your brain is spinning so intensely that fainting seems inevitable. Now, say, "Good morning," to one who may suffer from a stress-related illness.*

*Every day, people attempt to function normally, although many find themselves plagued with these types of stress-induced symptoms. It can even become worse, for, as one experiences these symptoms, a feeling of panic may arise concerning the severity and cause of such symptoms. This panic may eventually lead to a debilitating fear of the symptoms. A pervading sense of helplessness/hopelessness and worry is then added to an already painful situation of physical and mental torment. This feeling of helplessness and hopelessness often leads to depression. It does not take long for stress to blossom into physical symptoms, then panic or fear of the symptoms, and, then, depressive symptoms. The domino-effect of symptoms continues and intensifies.*

*I was, of course, examined by several medical doctors who sought to find a cause to my weakening condition. But, after a battery of painful, frustrating, and costly tests, no cause could be found! No tumors, no viruses, no cancerous tissues, no hidden infections, no ulcers, no eyesight problems, no nothing. I was "fine." What on earth could be causing these debilitating symptoms? Stress was never suggested as a possible cause, nor would I have believed it could cause such problems. What did I have to be stressed about except these ridiculous symptoms?!!*

*Living in this pitiful existence, while being a college student, did not help me achieve my academic and athletic goals. In fact, I felt even the simplest demands on my schedule becoming too much for me; a constant state of exhaustion encompassed my body. The "sickness," as I called it, was destroying me.*

*Then, while on summer break from school, I talked with a friend's mom, who happened to be a nurse, and her husband, who happened to be a physician. I explained to them my continually weakening state, and they mentioned it might be a stress-related illness. I said to myself, Stress? Isn't that for 45-year-old CEO's who have a family, unpaid bills, long hours at work, a poor diet, get little sleep, etc.? However, after a bit more thought, it seemed that those characteristics, in fact, applied to this 20-year-old college student, as well. I decided to see the Clinical Nurse Specialist. Besides, there was nowhere else to turn, except counseling. Every other route of investigation had been explored, and all had turned up nothing. Basically, I was just so sick of being sick that I was ready to try anything. The decision to see a stress-related illness specialist would change my life.*

*I met with Dr. Lyon only six times. It did not take long for me to realize that I had accumulated a ton of stressful baggage from the past, and that, in the present, I had even more stress being added to my system daily. The first step in my recovery came through simply identifying some very stressful situations in my life. These included leaving my support system of friends behind when I went out of state to college and feeling a loss of my spiritual self and, as a result, losing meaning or purpose in my life. I was, then, shown that thoughts really do cause feelings and that distortion and negativity of even the smallest thought can build up through similar thoughts and cause one overall sickening feeling. I identified new thoughts and counter-thoughts to focus on and practice. I began to think differently, that is, I made a conscious effort to control and limit the amount of negative thoughts I had. If I was in a situation and began focusing on negative aspects, I, then, focused my mind on positive aspects of situations. If I felt myself troubled or disturbed, I would recognize and focus on some of the positive aspects of my life. Obviously, you cannot just pretend that your problems do not exist. But, the focus of your thought can eliminate stress. Stress is a feeling, just like loving, or hating, and it, too, is triggered by thoughts. Thus, it is thoughts which control stress. It may sound like a mental game since your problems are not likely to disappear, but, ultimately, it is the mind that creates the worse problems. And, it is the mind that can be helped by these techniques. It really amazed me how much limiting my negative thoughts helped me feel better.*

*The physical symptoms did not cease immediately, but a few more helpful techniques quickly ended their dominating hold on my life. When the symptoms would come on, I was taught to take a deep breath from the diaphragm and accept the symptom. I quit trying to fight the symptom. Instead, I welcomed it and tried to make it more intense! If it lingered, I would just go about my business, accepting it as I went along, and, within seconds, the symptom would leave. The real key came in accepting the symptom and not trying to force it away or fight it. Every time I found myself in a stressful situation, I focused on taking a deep breath, focused on something positive, and accepted any symptom that came along. Amazingly, hardly a physical symptom would appear using these techniques. I learned these techniques in only three sessions. I was definitely feeling better and more confident in my recovery.*

*By the end of the last three sessions, I was managing/preventing stress much better through the elimination of repeated negative thoughts and gradually pulling myself out of the pit of despair by eliminating stress emotions and finding new meanings and purpose in my life. I overcame my sickness and my fear of being sick.*

*After our sessions, I desperately wanted to know why no one had suggested earlier that my illness might be stress-induced. More than a year of incapacitating sickness was healed in two short weeks! It seems that healthcare providers should be at least familiar with the possibility of stress-related illness. Unfortunately, a lot of money and time was wasted to no avail for me. Certainly, diseases need to be ruled out as a possible cause of a patient's symptoms, but why not also consider stress?*

*The bottom line is I learned that stress is not caused by external events. It is how we choose to perceive and interpret situations. I learned that difficult situations and stress are not the same thing! For those suffering from stress-related illnesses, there is hope. Stress emotions and stress-related physical symptoms can be eliminated by managing your thoughts. That feeling of helplessness/hopelessness can be exchanged for healthy confidence. I am fully aware that my six counseling sessions did not change my world, but it changed me – and that made all the difference!*

Craig's story is very powerful and demonstrates how stress emotions, and the experience of significant changes, accompanied by a tremendous sense of loss, particularly in spiritual self, can contribute to chronic stress and stress-related illness. It's pretty amazing what he learned in a short period of time! As a postscript, after graduating from his undergrad program, he finished a master's degree and a PhD in his discipline and is a professor at a prestigious university.

Craig's grief work was particularly difficult because he felt lost and experienced anxiety growing into panic attacks. After he was able to eliminate the debilitating panic attacks, he was able, over time, to establish new patterns of meaning and a new purpose. Craig is now married, has two children, and enjoys life in a very successful academic career. He is *paying it forward* by helping others through his work!

## SITUATIONAL DEPRESSION

Situational depression is a short-term, stress-related type of depression. It differs from clinical depression in that it is experienced only briefly and can be eliminated without psychotropic drugs. Situational depression is commonly triggered by a significant life event such as the breakup of an important relationship, a job layoff, a diagnosis of a life-threatening disease, the death of a loved one, the loss of a pension, or retirement from a passionately-loved career with no additional purpose.[6] The break in continuity is what makes situational depression a fairly common occurrence in the grief experience.

Situational depression is frequently experienced as a sense of hopelessness, a lack of engagement in social relationships, trouble focusing, loss of appetite, insomnia, and difficulty concentrating. It becomes challenging to carry out usual daily activities. In fact, it might be difficult to get up in the morning and face the day.

A very important point, here, is that, although situational depression will often have an element of sadness, sadness and depression are not the same phenomena. It's often difficult to distinguish between sadness and situational depression. Remember, sadness is not a stress emotion.

In my experience with clients, there are three common themes that contribute to situational depression after a traumatic event or loss. It appears that people who do not allow themselves to get caught up into these three themes do not experience situational depression after a traumatic event.

The first theme that contributes to situational depression is unrelenting, chronic anger, that is, experiencing anger because what happened was not expected. *It's just not fair! It's not right!* You dwell on what happened and how it used to be. The second theme is blaming yourself for what happened. *I should have known that it was possible to lose my pension. I should have known that I needed to diversify my investments.* Remember, expecting yourself to control others, or to control the uncontrollable, is fertile ground for unjustified guilt and, therefore, situational depression. The third theme is experiencing anxiety (because you focus on the future and imagine all kinds of additional negative consequences). I would frequently share with clients that the perfect recipe for situational depression after a traumatic event is 1/3 cup of anger, 1/3 cup of guilt, 1/3 cup of anxiety. This might be a very simplistic explanation, but it always made sense to clients.

Eliminating situational depression is not complicated, but that does not mean it's easy. Each contributing emotion must be addressed. Anger, in the case of a traumatic event, really serves no productive purpose. Although it may feel empowering, initially, in the long run chronic anger only contributes to your suffering and drains the energy you have available to deal successfully with the circumstances. It's not possible to change what happened, but it is possible for you to not focus on it, to forgive when needed, and to find something positive on which to focus. Regarding anxiety, it's important to accept the event, not focus on additional negative consequences, view the future as positive potentials, use the Work of Worry Guide, use positive self-talk, and use problem-focusing coping strategies, along with your social supports. Avoid blaming yourself for what happened. There are always external factors that were unforeseeable and not controllable.

The experience of grief is a fact of life. Each of us, typically more than once in a lifetime, will experience grief. Grief work done well strengthens us. It teaches us important lessons in the realities of life and love.

## TIPS FOR WEATHERING THE GRIEF PROCESS AND AVOIDING SITUATIONAL DEPRESSION

1. Accept the sadness.

2. Allow yourself to experience the sadness and recognize that, although it's painful, it's also an affirmation of love.

3. Know that you'll need to take some risks in establishing new or revised patterns to discover what works and what doesn't work, what feels right, and what doesn't feel right – this is a type of adventure.

4. Be patient with yourself. Don't let frustration get in your way. It takes time to find your way to discover new patterns of being and doing and maybe even meaning or purpose.

5. Rather than feeling anxious and focusing on potential harm, focus on the potential for gain and that you'll discover something that really fits and feels right.

6. Avoid feeling guilty for something you didn't do. Recognize that things happen that we don't expect and that hindsight is 20/20 – you can learn from it but don't punish yourself.

7. Know that the discovery of what will work best for you is through trial and error, and that's ok.

## SUMMARY

Remember the grief process is work! Don't be surprised, while doing grief work, that you may feel tired or fatigued – that's normal. It requires a lot of effort to establish new patterns of thinking, doing, meaning, and purpose while also experiencing sadness and, perhaps, stress emotions. Establishing new patterns is often scary because you're venturing into the unknown, but, as we discussed in Chapter five, you can choose to view the experience as an adventure. To prevent situational depression, it's important to avoid dysfunctional anxiety, unjustified guilt, chronic anger, and getting frustrated. Be patient and kind to yourself while you're doing grief work. Express your sadness and experiences to those who care about and support you. Allow yourself to reflect on what was lost in a positive manner and how much what was lost meant to you. Although the sadness may never go away entirely, it does substantially reduce in intensity over time.

# EPILOGUE

**CONGRATULATIONS!** You now have the basic skills to effectively conquer stress. Being able to conquer stress on a day-to-day basis doesn't happen overnight. It takes practice and more practice by reflecting on your experiences and learning from them, but now you know what to work on. I often tell clients that your own reflective learning plays a central role in improving your stress conquering skills. When you're in a difficult situation and experience a stress-emotion, take some quiet time to ask yourself:

1. What is contributing to this difficult situation?

2. What internal and external demands are creating an overload?

3. What are the non-essential internal and external demands I can eliminate

4. Which resources could be helpful?

5. What stress emotion am I experiencing?

6. What belief or value is underlying my view of the situation?

7. What thought is triggering the emotion that needs to be changed?

Take time to reread chapters that are particularly relevant to your situation. **Learning to live stress-free is not one expedition, it is a *journey*! Yes, it takes effort. Be patient with yourself. You might take two steps forward and one step back, but, hey, you're already one step ahead. You *can* do it!**

On the next three pages, I've prepared a condensed version of *Haven't You Suffered Enough?*

TIPS to prevent and eliminate stress. This will be a helpful reference guide for you.

# TIPS TO PREVENT AND ELIMINATE STRESS

(You have my permission to copy these two pages to use as a reminder for *your personal use*.)

**Wake up in the morning *deciding*: I'm going to make it a good day!** I will not allow anything or anybody to steal my JOY! **When you're overloaded, initiate your *Demand Management* mode.**

**Eliminate non-essential demands.** Unload non-essential internal demands (perfectionism, toxic self-talk – use thought stopping, situational toxic thoughts, irrational rules) and external demands (set limits, say no, delegate, hold realistic expectations).

**Manage essential demands.** Delay what you can and /or delegate what you can. Don't try to do everything yourself. *Ask for help when you need it!* Don't expect that someone else will do it just the way you would . . . good enough *is* good enough!

**Maximize your resources.** Enhance your internal resources. Nurture your self-esteem — be kind to yourself. Nurture and encourage yourself. Allow time to recharge your batteries and maintain a good energy level. Use problem-focused coping strategies to deal with difficult situations. Use emotion-focused coping strategies when your problem-focused strategies are not working or you need to decrease the intensity of a stress-emotion to think more clearly. Avoid blaming and indulging. Enhance your external resources. Identify reliable sources of information. Pay attention to and nurture your circle of family, friends, and colleagues.

**Accept situations that you cannot control.** Trying to change things and situations that you cannot control is a waste of energy and a root cause of situational depression. A better strategy is to accept those situations and work around them, develop contingency plans, and/or go with the flow.

**View difficult situations as challenges or opportunities to learn.** Use adventure thinking and focus on what you will learn from the experience. Focus on something positive in difficult situations. Use positive situational focusing (PSF). You can find something positive in every difficult situation. Difficult situations and stress are *not* the same thing!

**Avoid dysfunctional anxiety.** Focus on the present! Take deep diaphragmatic breaths. Initiate problem-solving – the work of worry when anticipating a harm/loss. The work of worry eliminates anxiety when your concerns don't have a reasonable chance of happening and/or helps you constructively prevent or lessen or deal with actual harms/loses.

**Avoid unjustified guilt.** Avoid idealistic (unreachable) expectations of yourself – or 'shoulds' as they result in unjustified guilt. It is *not* possible to be your ideal in situations that are not ideal.

**Avoid chronic anger.** Set realistic expectations of others. Let go of unrealistic (not going to be met) expectations of others.

**Avoid frustration.** Set realistic goals using the REAP principles. Break large complex goals down into smaller accomplishable steps or tasks.

**Plan ahead yet take things a day at a time or a task at a time.** Being present limits your focus to the now of what needs to be done, which maximizes your effectiveness on the task at hand.

**Manage your environment.** Find a system of organization that works for you and use it! It's tough to function in chaos. Chaos contributes to feeling out-of-control and wastes time. *Also*, choose to be around or influenced by people that you enjoy – who uplift you. Avoid naysayers and chronic complainers as much as possible.

**Attend to your spiritual self** in whatever way works for you.

**Maintain a sense of humor.** Choose to be around people who can laugh. Create humorous experiences by reading humorous literature or watching humorous shows. Laugh a lot!

**Allow yourself to grieve.** Accept that any significant loss can trigger a complex of grief emotions. Allow yourself to be sad as it is a reminder of the importance of what was lost. Be patient with yourself as you explore establishing new or revised patterns of thinking, feeling, and doing.

**Maintain a grateful attitude.** Every morning, think about what you're grateful for . . . you can't feel grateful and stressed at the same time!

## Haven't You Suffered Enough?
By: Brenda L. Lyon PhD, CNS, RN
©2020

# REFERENCES

## INTRODUCTION

1. Lazarus, R. (1966). *Psychological stress and the coping Process*. New York, NY: McGraw-Hill Book Co.
2. Blair, J. (1987). *Who gets Sick: Thinking and health*. Houston: Peak Press.
3. Lyon, B.L., 1990. Getting back on track: Nursing's autonomous scope of practice, pp 267-274. N. Chaska (Ed.). *The Nursing Profession: Turning Points*
4. Dolbin, C., Smith, S., and Steinhardt, M.A. (2007). Relationships of factors to stress symptoms of illness. *American Journal of Health Behavior*, 31(4), 423-433.
5. Cousins, N., (1979). *Anatomy of an illness as perceived by the patient*. New York: W.W. Norton & Company.
6. Sobel, G. (1995). Rethinking medicine: Improving health outcomes with cost-effective psychosocial interventions. *Psychosomatic Medicine, 57*, 234-244.
7. Barsky, A.J., Orav, E.J., and Bates, D.W. (2005). Somatization increases medical utilization and costs independent of psychiatric and medical comorbidity. *Archives of General Psychiatry*, 62, 903-910.
8. Agency for Healthcare Research and Quality. (2008, April). *Mental health woes remain one of the top reasons for doctor visits*. Retrieved from http://www.ahrq.gov/research/apr08/0408RA33.htm on June 15, 2008.

9. Barsky, A.J., Orav, E.J., and Bates, D.W. (2005). Somatization increases medical utilization and costs independent of psychiatric and medical comorbidity. *Archives of General Psychiatry, 62*, 903-910.

10. Lyon, B.L., 1990. Getting back on track: Nursing's autonomous scope of practice, pp 267-274. In N. Chaska (Ed.). *The Nursing Profession: Turning Points*

11. Lyon, B.L., 1990. Getting back on track: Nursing's autonomous scope of practice, pp 267-274. In N. Chaska (Ed.). *The Nursing Profession: Turning Points*

## CHAPTER 1: RETHINKING STRESS

1. Selye, H. (1973). The evolution of the stress concept. *American Scientist, 61*, 692-699.

2. Selye, H. (1976). *The stress of life.* 2nd Ed. *New York, NY: McGraw-Hill Book Co.*

3. Lyon, B.L. and Werner, J. (1987). Stress. In Fitzpatick, J. & R.L. Taunton (Eds.). *Annual Review of Nursing Research. 5*, 3-22. New York: Springer.

4. Mason, J.W. (1971), A re-evaluation of the concept of "non-specificity" in stress theory. *Journal of Psychiatric Research, 8*, 323-333.

5. Mason, J.W. (1975). A historical view of the stress field. Part I. *Journal of Human Stress*, 6-12.

6. Mason, J.W. (1975). A historical view of the stress field. Part II. *Journal of Human Stress*, 22-36.

7. Lyon, B.L. and Werner, J. (1987). Stress. In Fitzpatick, J. & R.L. Taunton (Eds.). *Annual Review of Nursing Research. 5*, 3-22. New York: Springer.

8. Selye, H. (1976). Forty years of stress research: Principle remaining problems and misconceptions. *Canadian Medical Association Journal, 115*, 53-55.

9. Holmes, T.H. & Rahe, R.H. (1967). The social readjustment rating scale. *Journal of Psychosomatic Research, 11*:213-218.

10. Rahe, R.H. & Arthur, R.J. (1978). Life changes and illness studies: Past history and future directions. *Journal of Human Stress*, 3-15.

11. Rahe, R.H. (1974). The pathway between subjects' recent life changes and their near-future illness reports. In B. Dohrenwend & B. Dohrenwend (Eds.), *Stressful life events: Their nature and effects* (pp. 73-86). NY: Wiley.

12. Kobasa, S. (1979). Stressful life events, personality, and health: An inquiry into hardiness. *Journal of Personality and Social Psychology, 37,* 1-11.

13. Kobasa, S. (1982). Hardiness and health: A prospective study. *Journal of Personality and Social Psychology, 42*(1), 168-177.

14. Sarason, I.G., Johnson, J.H., and Siegel, J. M. (1978). Assessing the Impact of Life Changes: Development of the Life Experiences Survey. *Journal of Consulting and Clinical Psychology, 46*(5), 932-946,

15. Lazarus, R. (1966). *Psychological stress and the coping Process.* New York, NY: McGraw-Hill Book Co.

16. Lazarus, R. and Folkman, S. (1984). *Stress, appraisal and coping.* New York, N.Y., Springer.

17. Lazarus, R. (1966). *Psychological stress and the coping Process.* New York, NY: McGraw-Hill Book Co.

18. Lazarus, R. and Folkman, S. (1984). *Stress, appraisal and coping.* New York, N.Y., Springer.

19. Wallston, K.A., Wallston, B.S., Smith, S., and Dobbins, C. (1987). Perceived control and health. *Current Psychology, 6*(1), 5-25.

20. Lazarus, R. (2000). Evolution of a model of stress, coping, and discrete emotions. In V.H. Rice (Ed.), *Handbook of stress, coping and health: Implications for nursing research, theory and practice.* 195-222. Thousand Oaks: Sage.

21. Rokeach, M. (1968). *Beliefs, attitudes and values: A theory of organization and change.* San Francisco, CA: Jossey-Bass.

22. Rokeach, M. (1973). *The nature of human values.* New York: The Free Press.

## CHAPTER 2: WHEN DEMANDS AND RESOURCES ARE OUT OF BALANCE

1. Lyon, B. (1987). *Stress management: An essential ingredient for good health.* Indianapolis: Health Potentials Unlimited.
2. Lyon, B.L. (2002). Cognitive self-care skills: A model for managing stressful lifestyles. *The Nursing Clinics of North America,* 37(2):285-294.

## CHAPTER 3: ELIMINATING NON-ESSENTIAL DEMANDS

1. Van Gemert, L. (2017). *Perfectionism: A practical guide to managing "never good enough,* Tucson, Arizona: Great Potential Press.
2. Van Gemert, L. (2017). *Perfectionism: A practical guide to managing "never good enough,* Tucson, Arizona: Great Potential Press.
3. Beck, A. T. (1979). *Cognitive therapy and the emotion disorders.* New York, N.Y.: International Universities Press.
4. McKay, M, Davis, M, and Fanning, P. (1997). *Thoughts and feelings: Taking control of your moods and your life.* Oakland, CA: New Harbinger Publications, Inc.
5. Beck, A. T. (1979). *Cognitive therapy and the emotion disorders.* New York, N.Y.: International Universities Press.
6. McKay, M, Davis, M, and Fanning, P. (1997). *Thoughts and feelings: Taking control of your moods and your life.* Oakland, CA: New Harbinger Publications, Inc.
7. Allen, J (2010). *As a man thinketh.* USA: www. Best Success. Net
8. Todd, D., Hardy, J. and Oliver, E. (2011). Effects of self-talk: A systematic review. *Journal of Sport and Exercise Psychology, 33*(5): 666-87.
9. McKay, M. and Fanning, P ( 2000). *Self-esteem.* Oakland, CA: New Harbinger Publications.
10. Wallston, K.A., Wallston, B.S., Smith, S., and Dobbins, C. (1987). Perceived control and health. *Current Psychology*, 6(1), 5-25.
11. McKay, M, Davis, M, and Fanning, P. (1997). *Thoughts and feelings: Taking control of your moods and your life.* Oakland, CA: New Harbinger Publications, Inc.

12. Smith, M.M., 1986. *When I say no, I feel guilty.* New York: Bantam Books.

## CHAPTER 4: MAXIMIZING RESOURCES

1. Branden, N. (1988). *How to raise your self-esteem: The proven action-oriented approach to greater self-respect and self-confidence.* New York, N.Y.: Random House.

2. Branden, N. (1995). *Six pillars of self-esteem.* New York, N.Y.: Random House.

3. Savarese, G., Carpinelli, L., Fasono, O., Mollo, M., Pecoraro, N., and Iannascone, A. (2013). Study of correlation between self-esteem, coping and clinical symptoms in a group of young adults. *European Scientific Journal, 9*(29), 1857-1871.

4. Lazarus, R. (1966). *Psychological stress and the coping process.* New York, NY: McGraw-Hill Book Co.

5. Lazarus, R. and Folkman, S. (1984). *Stress, appraisal and coping.* New York, N.Y., Springer.

6. Lazarus, R. (1966). *Psychological stress and the coping process.* New York, NY: McGraw-Hill Book Co.

7. Lazarus, R. and Folkman, S. (1984). *Stress, appraisal and coping.* New York, N.Y., Springer.

8. Folkman, S. (1997). Positive psychological states and coping with severe stress. *Social Science Medicine.* 45(3), 207-221.

9. Koenig, H.G., McCullough, M.E., Larson, D.B. (2001*). Handbook of religion and health.* Oxford: Oxford University Press.

10. Koenig, H.G. (2004). Religion, spirituality, and medicine: Research findings and implication for clinical practice. *Southern Medical Journal*, 97(12): 1194-1200.

11. Pargament, K.I. (1997). *The psychology of religion and coping.* New York: Guilford.

12. Levine, M. (2008). Prayer as coping: A psychological analysis. *Journal of Health Care Chaplaincy*, 15(2), 80-98.

13. Lyon, B.L. (2002). Social support as TLC: The great elixir. *Reflections in Nursing Leadership, 27*(4), 36-37, 51.

14. Underwood, P. (2000). Social support: The promise and the reality (pp.376-391). In Rice, V. (Ed.). *Handbook of stress, coping and health: Implications for Nursing Research, Theory, and Practice.* Thousand Oaks, CA: Sage Publications, Inc.

## CHAPTER 5: HOW YOU PERCEIVE DIFFICULT SITUATIONS

1. Lazarus, R. (1966). *Psychological stress and the coping Process.* New York, NY: McGraw-Hill Book Co.

2. Lazarus, R., and Folkman, S. (1984). *Stress, appraisal, and coping.* New York, Springer Publishing Co.

3. Lazarus, R., and Folkman, S. (1984). *Stress, appraisal, and coping.* New York, Springer Publishing Co.

4. Lyon, B.L. (2001). Strategies to enhance positive situational focusing skills. *Reflections in Nursing Leadership, 27*(3), 36-37, 44.

5. Lyon, B.L. (2001). Positive situational focusing: Pollyanna or a powerful stress prevention strategy? *Reflections in Nursing Leadership, 27*(2), 38-39,45.

6. Watson, D. and Pennebaker, J.W. (1989). Health complaints, stress and distress: Exploring the central role of negative affectivity. *Psychological Review, 96*, 234-254.

7. Peal, N.V. (1952). *The power of positive thinking: A practical guide to mastering the problems of everyday living.* New York, N.Y.: Prentice-Hall, Inc.

8. Steptoe, A, Dockray, S., and Wardle, J. (2009). Positive affect and psychobiological processes relevant to health, *Journal of Personality, 77*(6), 1747-2886.

9. Hanson, R. (2013). *Hardwiring happiness: The new brain science of contentment, calm and confidence.* New York, N.Y.: Random House, LLC.

10. Allen, J. (1989). <u>*As a man thinketh*</u>. Philadelphia: Running Press.

11. Morin, A. (2014). 7 scientifically proven benefits of gratitude that will motivate you to give thanks year-round. Forbes Magazine, 11/, 23

12. Christie, W., and Moore, C. (2005). The impact of humor on patients with cancer. *Clinical Journal of Oncology Nursing, 9*(2):211-216.

13. Fritz, H.L., Russek, L.M., Dillon, M.M. (2017). Humor use moderates the relation of stressful life events with psychological distress. *Personality and Social Psychology Bulletin, 43*(6): 845-859.

14. Bennett, A.P., and Lengasher, C. (2007). Humor and laughter may influence health: III. Laughter and health outcomes, *Evidence-based Complementary and Alternative Medicine, 5*(1): 37-40.

15. Carlson, R. (1993). *You can feel good again: Common sense strategies for releasing unhappiness and changing your life.* New York, NY: Plume Press.

## CHAPTER 6: CONQUERING DYSFUNCTIONAL ANXIETY

1. Lyon, B.L. (2000). Conquering dysfunctional anxiety. *Reflections in Nursing Leadership, 26*(4), 33-35,45.

2. Donald, J.N., Atkins, P.W.B., Parker, P.D., Christie, A.M., and Ryan, R.M. (2016). Daily stress and the benefits of mindfulness: Examining the daily and longitudinal relations between present-moment awareness and stress response. *Journal of Personality, (65),* 30-27.

3. Goyal, M., Singh, S., Sibinger, S. (2014). Meditation programs for psychological stress and well-being. *Journal of the American Medical Association (JAMA), 174*(3), 357-368.

4. Lyon, B. L. (2001). Work of worry guide. *Reflections on Nursing Leadership, 27*(1):26.

5. Janis, I. (1958). *Psychological stress: Psychoanalytic and behavioral studies of surgical patients.* New York: Wiley.

6. Mathew, G. and Wells, A. (2000). Attention, automaticity, and affective disorder. *Behavior Modification, 24*(1), 69-93.

7. Benson, H. (1975). *The relaxation response.* New York. Harper Collins Publishing.

8.  Dusek, J.A. and Benson, H. (2009). Mind-body medicine. *Minnesota Medicine, 82*(5): 47-50.

9.  Weeks, C., 1990. *Hope and help for your nerves.* New York: Signet.

10. Weeks, C., 1990. *Hope and help for your nerves.* New York: Signet.

## CHAPTER 7: CONQUERING UNJUSTIFIED GUILT

1.  Lyon, B.L. (2000). Conquering stress. *Reflections in Nursing Leadership, 26*(1), 22-23, 43.

2.  Rokeach, M. (1968). *Beliefs, attitudes and values: A theory of organization and change.* San Francisco, CA: Jossey-Bass.

3.  Rokeach, M. (1973). *The nature of human values.* New York: The Free Press.

4.  Tangney, J.P., Miller, R.S., Flicker, L. & Barlow, D.H. (1996). Are shame, guilt and embarrassment distinct emotions? *Journal of Personality and Social Psychology, 70*(60), 1256-1264.

5.  Weiner, B. (1974). *Achievement motivation and attribution theory.* Morristown, N.J.: General Learning Press.

6.  Lyon, B. (2000). Conquering stress. *Reflections in Nursing Leadership, 26(1), 22-23, 43.*

## CHAPTER 8: CONQUERING CHRONIC ANGER

1.  National Institute for the Clinical Application of Behavioral Medicine (NICABM), (2017). How anger affects your brain and body. Accessed 2/17/2019, https://www.iahe.com>docs>articles.

2.  Snyder, M. and Stokas, A.A. (1999). Interpersonal processes: The interplay of cognitive, motivational and behavioral activities in social interaction, *Annual Review of Psychology, 50,* 273-303.

3.  Scott, E. (2006). Reduce stress with increased assertiveness. Accessed at http://stress.about.com/od/relationships/p/profileassertiv.htm on July 1, 2011.

4. Woodham-Smith, (1950*). Florence Nightingale.* London: Constable & Company.

5. Scott, E. (2007). Learn assertive communication in five easy steps. Accessed at http://stress.about.com/od/relationships/ht/how to assert. htm on July 1, 2011.

6. Lyon, B.L. (2000). *Conquering chronic anger. Reflections in Nursing Leadership, 26*(2), 30-31, 45.

7. Ellis, A. (1996). *Anger: How to live with and without it.* New York: Carol Publishing Group.

8. McKay, M., Roger, P., & McKay, J. (1989). *When anger hurts: Quieting the storm within.* Oakland, CA: New Harbinger Publications, Inc.

9. Potter-Efron, R. (1994). *Angry all the time: An emergency guide to anger control.* Oakland, CA: New Harbinger Publications, Inc.

10. Thomas, S. (1998). *Transforming nurses' anger and pain: Steps toward healing.* New York, NY: Springer Publishing Company, Inc.

11. Lyon, B.L. (2000). *Situational anger and self-empowerment. Reflections in Nursing Leadership, 26*(3), 36-39.

12. Ellis, A. (1996). *Anger: How to live with and without it.* New York: Carol Publishing Group.

13. Luskin, F. (2002). *Forgive for Good: A Proven Prescription for Health and Happiness.* San Francisco: Harper-Collins Publishers, Inc.

## CHAPTER 9: CONQUERING FRUSTRATION

1. Plutchik, R. (1991). *The Emotions.* University Press of America. Lanham, Maryland.

2. Lyon, B.L. (2001) Conquering frustration: REAPing the Benefits. *Reflections in Nursing Leadership, 27*(1), 38-37, 46.

# CHAPTER 10: DEALING WITH LOSS/GRIEF AND SITUATIONAL DEPRESSION

1. Kubler-Ross, E. and Byock, I. (2011). *On death and dying*. New York, N.Y.: Simon and Schuster, Inc.

2. Maciejowski, P.K., Zhang, B., Block, S.D., Pregerson, H.G. (2007). An empirical examination of the stages theory of grief. Journal of the American Medical Association. 297(7): 716-23.

3. Bonanno, G. (2009). The other side of sadness. What the new science of bereavement tells us about life after loss. Basic Books, New York, N.Y.

4. "Five fallacies of Grief: Debunking psychological stages." (2008). *Scientific American*. Retrieved November 15, 2018.

5. Marris, P. (1974). *Loss and change*. Pantheon Books. London, England.

6. Gronley, M. (2018). Types of depression. Scottsdale Mental Health Care, P.C. Accessed at pyschiatricscotsdale.com on July 7, 2018.

7. Stressdone, M. (2014). *Situational depression: How to feel better while dealing with situational depression*. Amazon Digital Services, LLC.

# ABOUT THE AUTHOR

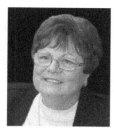 Dr. Brenda Lyon PhD, CNS, RN holds a bachelor's, master's and PhD in nursing from Indiana University. She was a professor at Indiana University School of Nursing for 39 years, teaching in the Master's and PhD programs. She is currently a Professor Emerita at the university.

Dr. Lyon, as a Clinical Nurse Specialist, had a private practice in stress and stress-related physical illness for over 34 years. She has conducted over 350 workshops for corporations, health professionals, and trade associations focused on helping people learn how to prevent and eliminate stress in their lives. She has published over 20 articles and contributed to four published books focused on stress and stress management and is also the author of the national award-winning *Conquering Stress* monograph and video series published by Glaxo-Smith Kline.

Dr. Lyon is a recipient of the Midwest Nursing Research Society's Distinguished Contribution to the Science of Stress and Coping Award by the Stress and Coping Research Section. She received Indiana University's prestigious W. George Pinnell Award for Outstanding Service nationally and in the field of stress and coping. She is a Fellow in both the American Academy of Nursing and in the interdisciplinary National Academies of Practice.

Brenda L. Lyon PhD, CNS, RN
Health Potentials Unlimited, LLC
Noblesville, Indiana
Copyright 2020